**Occupational
Therapy in
Long-term
Psychiatry**

For the staff and students of
Salford School of Occupational Therapy

Occupational Therapy in Long-term Psychiatry

Moya Willson
MSc TDip COT
Senior Lecturer, Salford School
of Occupational Therapy, Salford

SECOND EDITION

CHURCHILL LIVINGSTONE
EDINBURGH LONDON MELBOURNE AND NEW YORK 1987

CHURCHILL LIVINGSTONE
Medical Division of Longman Group UK Limited

Distributed in the United States of America by Churchill Livingstone Inc.,
650 Avenue of the Americas, New York, N.Y. 10011, and by associated companies,
branches and representatives throughout the world.

First edition 1983
Second edition 1987
    Reprinted 1989
    Reprinted 1992
    Reprinted 1993
    Reprinted 1995

ISBN 0-443-03565-2

British Library Cataloguing in Publication Data
A catalogue record for this book is available from the British Library

Library of Congress Cataloguing in Publication Data
A catalogue record for this book is available from the Library of Congress

The
publisher's
policy is to use
**paper manufactured
from sustainable forests**

Produced by Longman Singapore Publishers (Pte) Ltd.
Printed in Singapore

Preface to the Second Edition

This book has now been bought, and sometimes read, by three intakes of occupational therapy students.

Some have enjoyed it more than others and a few, to my delight, have made it their own with the addition of marginal comments and notes.

The second edition is intended to serve another few years of students in training who, I hope, should feel equally free to argue and develop the basic material. Few alterations have been made, not because it cannot be improved but because I do not enjoy tinkering. I have, however, acceded to the many requests to add a chapter on care in the community.

I am grateful to all those who have supported and used my work and hope that this edition will provide a friendly and uncomplicated guide to those yet to enter the maze of psychiatric practice.

Salford, 1987   Moya Willson

Preface to the First Edition

This book has been written primarily for occupational therapy students, and occupational therapists working with long-term psychiatric patients. I hope it may also be helpful to a wider range of colleagues in other fields whose principal concern is this group of patients, and to occupational therapists working in other areas of speciality.

It is difficult to define long-term psychiatric problems on the basis of diagnosis. The intention therefore has been to focus on the needs and treatment of those who, for any reason, experience institutional care as a way of life or who are sufficiently disabled to require repeated referral for treatment. This means that patients who require help only during specific crises in their lives, or who have acute problems which can be alleviated by treatment within a year or less, are not generally under consideration.

Psychiatric practice embraces a wide range of organic and social problems. The extent of this range is in part logical and in part historical. A discipline which concerns itself with psychotic disorders, mental handicap, responses to social stress, organic deficiencies and deterioration, variations in mood and personality, and developmental crises does not lend itself to any one approach to therapy. The book is therefore limited to concern for those patients with long-standing or permanently disabling problems where the major task is one of rehabilitation. This includes those with 'psychotic' disorders, the institutionalized, the elderly mentally infirm, and to an extent the mentally handicapped, if for no other reason than that these groups form the majority of patients under psychiatric care.

The first five chapters, constituting Part One, consider some of the theories and models of treatment which are relevant to occupational therapists working in this field. As far as possible I have tried not to assume too much knowledge of psychology or allied subjects so that the contents may be comprehensible to students at an early stage of training. The concepts involved are, however, complex and these chapters should be used to revise, clarify or support other study rather than to replace it. The main intention has been to relate available knowledge to the specific needs of occupational therapists. Providing some perspective for the theoretical concepts inevitably involves a degree of personal opinion. This usually implies that any interpretation is 'common sense' if you agree with the writer, and irritating if you do not. Opinion is unavoidable in an area where no approach has been proved to be effective to the exclusion of all others. After all, if there was one straightforward solution to all problems then psychiatric hospitals would not contain their present population of patients, or of struggling occupational therapists and other workers.

The later chapters, making up Part Two, are concerned with the structure of occupational therapy for individuals and groups of patients. It is necessary to recognise that some knowledge of the theory upon which treatment is based is important to every therapist, however practically orientated. Without such knowledge it is difficult to evaluate and to improve upon the service which is being provided or to devise alternative programmes of treatment.

Successive chapters consider assessment, goal setting, environments, activities involved in treatment, and finally, evaluation. Guidelines and alternatives have been provided in preference to solutions. This is in recognition that professional colleagues are both sensitive and compassionate and that they consider each patient as being unique.

Finally, a brief word on what this book is *not*. It is not a cookery book: I can't give you a recipe which, correctly applied, will resolve all the problems experienced by those with long standing psychiatric disorders. If I could then occupational therapy would be a technical process and not a professional concern. A member of any profession has to select, from available theoretical knowledge and experience, an approach which is most applicable to the problem, to design its application and evaluate its results.

Whilst writing this book I have been ill-humoured, preoccupied and intolerant. My friends, colleagues and students have responded by being helpful, understanding and faithful. For this phenomenon I am grateful and extend my thanks to all those who have advised, criticised and encouraged me, in particular to Gavin and Averil Stewart and Diana Grellier, who read the manuscript, and Sue Ensor, who typed it.

Salford, 1983   Moya Willson

Contents

PART TWO   The structure of therapy

PART | **ONE**

Theories and
models of
treatment

1

Treatment based on theories of learning

The way in which people learn, and the ways in which behaviour is perpetuated, are of particular interest to those who are concerned with the care of long-term patients. Much of a therapist's time is spent in teaching people to perform tasks which will be useful to them, or in helping them to replace ineffective or unacceptable behaviour with more successful strategies.

The information given in this chapter is a brief, historical summary of some of the theories and techniques of learning which underlie these methods of treatment. For this and similar chapters in Part One, students should refer to the recommended reading lists at the end of each chapter for additional, more comprehensive information.

BEHAVIOURAL MODELS IN PSYCHIATRY

The premise

The term 'model', in psychiatry as in everyday usage, refers to a simplified representation of reality. The behavioural model in psychiatry explains or represents human behaviour in terms of learning: a person who is unable to function normally has either failed to learn or has adopted socially

3

unacceptable behaviour or behaviour which fails to achieve the appropriate goals.

Human behaviour embraces an endless range of skills and functions. Everything that an individual can be observed as doing is termed 'observable behaviour'. In seeing, hearing or feeling the activity of another person we are constantly experiencing their behaviour. There are certain aspects of a person, for example his mood, which cannot be observed directly but can only be inferred from behaviour such as smiling, crying, remaining silent, or the content of his speech. Observable behaviour normally includes the acquisition and use of language, the performance of tasks and the way in which an individual interacts with other people and with his environment. Psychologists of the behavioural school maintain that each of these behaviours is the result of learning. A combination of learnt behaviours directs the personality of the individual and his habitual manner of perceiving and participating in activities or relationships.

Since, according to the behaviourist, an inability to cope with the demands and activities of each day is due either to failure to learn, or to having learnt inadequate or inappropriate behaviours, a behavioural model of treatment involves identifying maladaptive behaviours and seeking to correct these by applying the principles of learning. This will involve both the elimination of some behaviours and the teaching of others. The behaviour itself is seen as the central problem rather than as an expression, or symptom, of less apparent emotional conflicts.

An example of faulty learning giving rise to psychological dysfunction can be seen in a patient who is habitually withdrawn, unable to sustain normal conversation and alarmed by being with a group of other people. His behavioural deficits may cause him to become isolated and to develop symptoms of anxiety or depression. However, if he can be taught a repertoire of social behaviour which enables him to communicate with others in a satisfying way then his confidence should increase and he may become a more sociable and able person. In this case maladaptive behaviour can be seen as a primary cause of psychological disorder.

In the above example the behavioural explanation of dysfunction is demonstrated and treatment clearly can be based on behavioural principles. Behavioural treatment is not, however, limited in its application to patients who have primary problems stemming from learning.

A majority of patients who have spent long periods of time within institutions lack both social skills and the ability to carry out normal tasks independently. Some, for example the mentally handicapped, may never have learnt these skills. Others may have lost previously acquired skills due to their *illness* or to their environment. Behavioural problems for these patients may be secondary but treatment based on theories of learning can still be the most appropriate. The behavioural therapies may not provide a remedy for the symptoms of schizophrenia but they might be instrumental in enabling the schizophrenic patient to live independently.

The terminology

Some brief definitions of key words are given here. This arrangement is based on the experience that a glossary discovered at the end of a topic is invariably too late.

Adaptive behaviour. Behaviour which is both effective and appropriate to the situation in which it is used. This term is preferable to the alternatives of 'good' and 'acceptable'. Both of these imply a subjective judgement on the part of the therapist. Adaptive behaviour should not only be socially acceptable but should work to the advantage of the subject.

Maladaptive behaviour. Behaviour which is either socially unacceptable or which fails to achieve the subject's goals. For example, reaching the front of the queue in a bank by producing a firearm is effective but unacceptable. Being too timid to object to unfair treatment is relatively acceptable but ineffective.

Positive reinforcement. A consequence of behaviour which the subject experiences as being rewarding. The obvious examples are material rewards such as food or money and social rewards such as praise or approval. Whether the reinforcement is positive or not depends on what the subject wanted whilst engaged in the behaviour. Being scolded or actively punished may be a positive reinforcement if the desire was for attention of any kind. Essentially a positive reinforcement is any consequence which makes it more likely that the causal behaviour will be repeated.

Negative reinforcement. A consequence which will cause the behaviour to be less likely to be repeated. In this sense negative reinforcement may simply be the absence of positive reinforcement, for example being ignored rather than either comforted or scolded. Sometimes it is important to identify factors which are currently inhibiting desired action, negative reinforcement may refer to the removal of an unpleasant stimulus in order to facilitate a desired behaviour.

Punishment. This is not the same as negative reinforcement. However, a punishment may discourage the repetition of a behaviour when it is experienced as a totally undesirable consequence.

Extrinsic reinforcement. A reinforcement which primarily is given or controlled by another person. This may be in the form of a tangible reward or of active social reinforcement such as praise or affection.

Intrinsic reinforcement. A consequence experienced internally by the subject without requiring the intervention of another person. Examples could include a personal sense of achievement or a feeling of belonging to or being accepted by a group of people. It is quite possible to describe intrinsic negative reinforcement such as guilt, self-disgust or anxiety.

Baseline behaviour. The pattern of behaviour emitted by the subject before treatment is commenced. When a maladaptive behaviour has been identified a baseline is constructed showing its frequency, duration, precipitating factors and usual consequences.

Extinction. A fading or disappearance of a behaviour due to lack of positive reinforcement.

THEORIES OF LEARNING

The mechanisms of learning and the conditions under which it takes place are the subjects of an abundance of psychological research and publication. In selecting and briefly describing a few topics of particular relevance to the practising therapist, there is a danger of implying that it is not necessary to appreciate the wider span of knowledge available. This would be as undesirable as the alternative danger of becoming entirely occupied by the efficiency of rats and pigeons, and the salivation of dogs, to the detriment of discussion related to the care of patients. Again, students are referred to the lists of recommended reading.

The theoretical concepts which need to be given emphasis by inclusion here are those of classical and instrumental conditioning, motivation, reinforcement and studies which may help a therapist in establishing an optimum environment for learning to take place.

Classical and instrumental conditioning

Classical conditioning

It would be difficult to discuss classical conditioning without looking to the work of Ivan Pavlov (1849–1936). To Pavlov all behaviour is reflexive in character. A simple reflex action such as blinking when poked in the eye or salivating at the sight or smell of appetizing food is a straightforward stimulus-response mechanism. In both these cases the stimulus and the response are unconditioned, that is, they have not had to be learnt. Pavlov considered that all forms of acquired behaviour are an extension of this basic reflex and are a result of conditioning. A previously 'neutral' stimulus when paired with an unconditioned stimulus becomes associated with the same response. Thus, in the simplest of his famous experiments, the previously 'neutral' stimulus of the bell is paired with the unconditioned stimulus of the meat powder to which the dog responds by salivating. After a number of trials the dog begins to salivate at the sound of the bell. The bell has therefore become a conditioned stimulus and the salivation a conditioned response.

Instrumental conditioning

As proposed by B. F. Skinner, this conditioning involves the animal in some kind of voluntary activity in order to gain reinforcement. A rat can be trained to press a lever in order to obtain a pellet of food. During training the naive rat may first of all step on the lever accidentally as one of many random behaviours emitted. The magazine which delivers food is operated by this chance behaviour. A second pressing of the lever may follow with less delay and time intervals continue to decrease until the rat is employed full time in operating the lever and eating the reinforcement. Two principles are involved: firstly, that the subject's voluntary behaviour is instrumental in obtaining the reinforcement; secondly, that the behaviour is contingent upon its outcome. Positive reinforcement increases the likelihood of a behaviour being repeated.

Classical conditioning and instrumental conditioning are two model which seek to explain the acquisition of behaviour. The debate is not, however, centred on whether one theory is more correct than the other but on whether or not there are two different types of learning. Assuming, for the moment, that there are two different types of learning it is convenient to term these respondent and operant.

Respondent learning

This appears to have close connections with classical conditioning. Respondent behaviours mainly involve responses of the autonomic nervous system and glandular secretions. Salivation, sweating and increased or decreased heart rate can all be called respondent behaviours. Several forms of treatment are based on respondent behaviour therapy: amongst these are systematic desensitization, assertiveness training, implosion and aversive conditioning. The work of J. Wolpe (1958) is of particular significance within these therapies. He developed techniques for the counter-conditioning of maladaptive behaviours. Such maladaptive behaviours include fear and anxiety towards situations which would normally be considered harmless. From research involving neurotic cats, he extended his study to the treatment of phobic humans.

The basic principle of counter-conditioning is the elimination of a maladaptive response by pairing it with a stronger incompatible response. This is known as *reciprocal inhibition*. For example, in the treatment of a simple phobia the symptoms of fear would be the maladaptive response and deep relaxation the incompatible response. Relaxation and fear cannot be experienced simultaneously. In order to give the incompatible response the advantage of relative strength, a hierarchy of anxiety-provoking situations would be prepared. Treatment progresses by confronting the patient with situations which gradually increase in their potential for inducing fear.

Operant learning

This is associated with instrumental conditioning. Operant behaviours involve voluntary movement or control on the part of the subject and skeletal or muscular action. A rat pressing a lever, a pigeon pecking at a disc and a human making a cup of tea are all operant behaviours. Treatment based on operant behaviour therapy include methods of shaping behaviour and 'token economies'. When the subject emits a behaviour, or an approximation towards a behaviour, which is desired by the therapist he is positively reinforced. Undesirable behaviour is extinguished by the absence of reinforcement.

Having used this categorization, it must be confessed that the distinctions between respondent and operant behaviours or therapies are not really as simple as all that. Some learning processes can be shown to involve both respondent and operant behaviours and it becomes a theoretical, if not a semantic, problem to disentangle them from each other. A second difficulty lies in the possibility of demonstrating the operant control of autonomic functions. This means that the premise of respondent behaviours being essentially visceral and operant behaviours skeletal does not really hold water. Miller (1969) and his associates have conducted a series of experiments to show that animals can learn to control the rate at which their hearts beat in order to gain reinforcement. Operant controls have also been established for temperature in different parts of the body, for localized changes in blood pressure, for stomach acidity and other functions. This indicates that people can be trained to exert voluntary control over such mechanisms within their own bodies. In order to achieve this some process of feedback is required and this is the basis of the bio-feedback techniques which are of growing interest within psychological medicine.

Despite this relevant digression the terms respondent and

operant are still useful tools in discussing behaviour and need not be entirely discarded.

Reinforcement and motivation

In a clinical setting it would be convenient and rather neat to be able to equate that most effective reinforcers with the primary physiological needs of food, water, oxygen, pain avoidance and sex. Unfortunately this does not appear to work for theoretical as well as for practical reasons. For example food and drink are sometimes used as reinforcers within a behaviour modification programme but prolonged deprivation is not ethical. There is also a considerable moral objection to the planned manipulation of pain. Whatever your ethical position, sex is inconvenient.

In theoretical terms there is insufficient evidence to show that human learning specifically requires primary reinforcement. Within a social learning framework it is incorrect to say that learning is brought about by reinforcement at all. Reinforcement is associated with motivation and not with the acquisition or change of behaviour by which we define learning. For example within a token economy scheme a patient may be positively reinforced by being given a token for making his own bed correctly. The giving of the token should make the patient more likely to repeat this behaviour but is not responsible for the patient's ability to understand or perform the necessary skills.

There are two ways of looking at secondary reinforcers. Firstly, their value is in a close association with primary reinforcers, for example money or tokens may be used to buy food. Secondly, it may be considered that secondary reinforcers have their own intrinsic value to the subject. Such reinforcers would include social approval, displays of affection, sweets, cigarettes or opportunities to participate in desired activities.

Studies of motivation include the drive-stimulus model proposed by Hull (1884–1952), theories related to reinforcement and to incentives, and more physiologically based investigations into the role of the ascending reticular activating system. These studies tend to concentrate on the relationship between motivation and primary physiological needs. There

have been experiments to show that animals are also motivated towards activity either for its own sake or by being
rewarded by opportunities to be further stimulated. For
example monkeys learn to press a lever in order to open a
window which they could look through (Butler, 1953) and will
also manipulate puzzles with no other reward than the finding
of a solution (Harlow et al, 1950).

But what about people? The motivations underlying human
activity appear to be much more complex and less understood. In addition to physiological needs a number of hierarchies of social and personal needs have been proposed.
The work of Abraham Maslow in this context will be discussed
within Chapter 2. Not only does motivation vary between
cultural groups but different individuals may perform the
same task for different reasons. One child may strive to excel
in a particular sport for his own satisfaction, another to please
an athletic parent and a third because he has been promised
some material reward.

Another most pertinent feature of man is his anticipatory
capacity. We look ahead to the eventual consequences of
present action. We know that if we spend our entire salary
cheque immediately on its receipt we will be uncomfortably
hard up before the next one arrives. We pay the electricity
bill, clean our teeth and our paint-brushes and put oil in the
car without immediate reinforcement. It is true that chained
learning can be demonstrated in animals. For example in
Wolfe's experiment monkeys learnt to press a lever in order
to obtain a poker chip which in turn could be inserted into
a vending machine in order to receive a grape. The monkeys
would continue to obtain and hoard poker chips for future
use when the grape vending machine was not available
(Wolfe, 1936). This behaviour seems slightly different,
however, from that of the student who refuses social engage-
ments in order to memorise the origins and insertions of all
the muscles of the upper limb in the hope of receiving a
qualification three years later.

In applying theories of learning to the behavioural treatment of patients the most appropriate reinforcement needs to
be chosen with care. Patients with long-standing depressive
symptoms or who have been diagnosed as being psychotically
ill may have a disturbance of volition arising from either

their condition or their environment. In practice this means that they will be more difficult to motivate that the rest of us who do not share these disadvantages. Any therapist with experience in long-term psychiatry will be familiar with this problem.

It is frequently necessary to base the early stages of treatment on a system of extrinsic reinforcement such as token economy because patients appear to lack a desire for social improvement or contact. The fact that cigarettes are often the most effective extrinsic positive reinforcement is a sad comment on the effects of institutional life. Encouraging patients to reinforce intrinsically their own behaviour by personal pride and satisfaction in social contact should be included and developed within any programme. This type of reinforcement is more natural and also longer lasting since successful behaviour does not depend on therapeutic control.

THE STRUCTURE OR BEHAVIOURAL TREATMENT

Organisation of treatment

Behavioural methods of treatment need to be ordered and consistent if they are to be effective. First one must establish who is to be involved in planning and carrying out the treatment. The patient is the central figure and should be involved as far as possible in formulating the behavioural goals and designing any programme. His co-operation is essential and it is much easier to co-operate if you understand what is going on.

Where principles of operant conditioning are being used it is important that reinforcement should be consistent. The same rules or consequences should be applied to the patient's behaviour in every context. For this reason the widest possible range of qualified or unqualified staff should be actively involved in treatment, or should be aware of its purpose. In some cases other patients may be involved in positively reinforcing, or ignoring, certain behaviours.

The processes involved in planning a structured treatment programme can be summarized as follows:

1. Identify maladaptive behaviour

Where behaviour is present which needs to be extinguished this should be defined as precisely as possible. Such behaviours may include aggressive outbursts, begging, attention seeking, social withdrawal and any other active or passive traits which are recognized as being maladaptive in the individual.

It is also important to be precise about deficits in behaviour. For example a general deficit in the maintenance of personal hygiene should be made more specific by listing skills which the patient does not possess such as cleaning teeth, looking after clothing or washing where and when appropriate. Other deficits may involve an inability to maintain accuracy at work or social contact at leisure.

2. Establish a baseline for treatment

This involves preparing, over a period of time, a record of the patient's behaviour before treatment commences. A recorded baseline should give information about the frequency of an identified behaviour, its duration, any precipitating events and its usual consequences. There are a number of ways of doing this and it is helpful to select the most appropriate.

Continuous observation is, of course, the most accurate, but staffing levels seldom permit it. In order to record a maladaptive habit such as rocking, withdrawing from social contact or irrelevant or antisocial speech, time sampling may be used. The patient is observed for a short period at regular intervals, for example five minutes in every hour. The resulting record of his behaviour during this time is used to formulate a picture of how and when the behaviour occurs over a few days.

Systematic recording may be appropriate for behaviours which occur as a spontaneous response. These might include aggressive outbursts, antisocial acts or, more positively, social contact and the use of initiative. Each relevant event is recorded by the member of staff most closely concerned with the patient at the time it occurs. Over a period these records combine to form a profile of the current pattern of behaviour. Where a certain behaviour is absent or never produced spontaneously the baseline can be assessed pretty rapidly as being nil.

3. Identification of adaptive behaviour

This is also known as establishing behavioural goals. It is important to be specific, as with maladaptive behaviours, in order to establish immediate and effective reinforcement. When a complex task is being taught, or when social skills are being developed, it is often necessary to break the target down into a series of progressive subsidiary goals. This allows the reinforcement of each stage in learning without having to wait until the entire behaviour has been achieved successfully.

A process of 'shaping' behaviour can be used when approximations towards the desired behaviour are reinforced. Thus, if the desired behaviour is that a patient should join with others in co-operative activity, he may be rewarded first for remaining in the same room, then for watching others participate and so on.

4. Identification of appropriate reinforcement

The necessity of selecting the most appropriate reinforcing agent has already been discussed. Positive reinforcement should be used whenever possible. It is important to decide not only on the nature of the reinforcement but also on its most appropriate administration.

To be most effective the consequence of a behaviour should follow without delay. To a child the distant promise of being sent to bed early, or of receiving a bigger Christmas present, is normally less effective than an immediate response whether pleasant or otherwise. Is the patient to be reinforced on every occasion that the produces the desired behaviour or will the system be one of partial, or intermittent, reinforcement? Reinforcement is equally, if not more, effective when given intermittently.

Intermittent reinforcement can be arranged in relation to time, that is a patient may be reinforced at intervals while he is involved in activity. If the time between reinforcements is regular this is known as a 'fixed interval schedule'. If reinforcement is random within time then it is described as being of 'variable interval'. It may be more appropriate to relate the reinforcement to the patient repeating a behaviour a number of times. If he is involved in a repetitive task and a set number of completed operations earns reinforcement, then this would be described as a 'fixed ratio'. More random reinforcement of repeated behaviours becomes, logically enough, a 'variable ratio' schedule.

5. Selection of the treatment method

There are numerous different methods of behavioural treatment just as there are lots of different recipes for making jam. The reasons for choosing a particular method, and the results, may be different but the basic principles remain constant. Modelling, token economies, contractural methods, desensitization, backward chaining and assertiveness or social skills training will be discussed below. These have been selected as being of particular significance to the occupational therapist. Other methods such as implosive or aversion therapy have fewer applications in this context, unless the therapist is so horrific in appearance or personality that the patient develops an aversion to all forms of prescribed activity.

6. Planning and carrying out the treatment

This process may seem rather far down the list but only becomes effectively possible after all the previous preparation has been done. There are two major concerns: that the programme should be systematic and that it should be consistent.

A well-devised programme should be recorded on paper and should answer the following questions:

1. During what part of the patient's day is the treatment programme in operation?
2. Who is the co-ordinator of this programme?
3. Apart from the patient and the co-ordinator, who else is involved and what part are they expected to play?
4. What activities will the patient be actively engaged in and when will these take place?

5. When will the effectiveness of the programme be evaluated so that any modifications or alternatives may be considered?

Techniques

Modelling

The theories of learning which have been described tend to depict behaviour as the result of directly experienced consequences. In fact we do not need to experience personally every situation in order to learn. There is an ability to learn vicariously by observing the performance or the coping behaviour of others. This capacity to learn by observation enables an individual to acquire quite complex patterns of behaviour without needing to resort to trial and error.

As a planned part of treatment the therapist may deliberately model appropriate behaviours for the patient to copy and later to rehearse. He is most likely to adopt these if he also observes that such behaviours command agreeable consequences. Even when the therapist is not deliberately modelling behaviour the patient naturally continues to observe and perhaps to learn. This means that in all contacts with patients and with colleagues, and in all instances of social interaction or problem solving, therapists need to remember that their own personal behaviour continues to be a part of the learning environment.

Systematic desensitization

The principles of desensitization have been described previously in the brief discussion of Wolpe's work on counter-conditioning. This form of treatment for anxiety is only used when the anxiety is inappropriate or has occurred as a result of conditioning. There are three main procedures:

1. Training the patient in methods of deep relaxation.
2. Constructing a hierarchy of anxiety-provoking situations.
3. Presenting the patient with these situations; progressing through the hierarchy whilst he is in a relaxed state.

The original form of desensitization requires patients to visualize items on the hierarchy during treatment sessions.

Problems arise either when the patient is unable to learn relaxation to an effective depth or when he is unable to visualize anxiety- provoking situations adequately. Real life desensitization may be more effective in such cases. This means that as far as possible the patient is presented with a hierarchy of actual situations.

The simplest examples to give are those relating to a specific phobia such as fear of dogs, heights or open spaces. Anxiety related to social environments may also be treated by real life exposure. It is in the execution of real life desensitization that the occupational therapist may be most closely involved in this method of treatment. Within the occupational therapy department relevant social situations may be devised, or materials and situations presented to the patient in hierarchical order, accompanied by both relaxation and encouragement. The occupational therapist may also be involved in arranging for the patient to venture outside the hospital. This may be required for the patient to reach a series of progressive goals as part of a programme to desensitize him to fears of going outside or of using transport or public facilities.

Desensitization may also be assisted by linking the treatment programme with modelling. The therapist models the confrontation of the feared situation either in real life or on a film or video. Allowing the patient to observe another individual coping with a threatening situation may serve as a useful adjunct to his own programme.

Token economy

A token economy is a systematic method of treatment whereby certain defined behaviours are given an extrinsic value. For example, punctuality, social contact or participation in activity are rewarded by the giving of tokens. Maladaptive behaviours may result in tokens being withdrawn. Tokens may be accumulated and used in exchange for food, tobacco, weekend leave, privileges or any other reward that the patient desires.

For this system to work the patient must understand what to do in order to gain the token, and the staff must be consistent in carrying out the programme. The system breaks down when the patient discovers that certain behaviours are reinforced in one setting but not in another, or that certain members of staff are a relatively 'soft touch'.

Such programmes may be devised in order to treat a group of patients, criteria for reinforcement of behaviour being similar for each individual. This is simpler to administer since a large range of staff may be able to comply, clearly understanding the token value of each adaptive behaviour. The disadvantages of a poorly designed programme include the encouragement of even greater passivity and concurrence on the part of the patients. After all, if such treatment methods were to be perfectly effective everyone would end up behaving in the same way. How you regard such as eventuality depends on your definition of normality.

A second approach to applying this technique is to set individual targets and token reward schedules for each patient. This should be more appropriate to individuals problems and more effective but is also more difficult to administer effectively. A visual record should be kept for the reference of both patient and staff. The patient may also carry a card which states his current target behaviours. A vital component of such treatments is continuous and relevant communication between the staff involved.

Contractual methods

A formal contract relating to behaviour and its consequences may be drawn up between the patient and the staff. This type of arrangement is similar in principle to token economy. Such a contract should state maladaptive behaviours on the part of the patient and the way in which staff will respond if such behaviours are produced. Adaptive behaviours or targets will also be defined and the consequences of these laid down.

Consider, for example, a patient who complains about his own situation continuously and who fails to reinforce others by responding verbally or otherwise to their conversation. His contract may state that, should he complain for more than a specified amount of time, no attention will be paid to him or privileges will be withdrawn. Should he demonstrate concern for others, or involvement with them, then he will gain attention or some other extrinsic reward.

Backward chaining

Many tasks can be broken down into a number of specific parts. Washing hair, for example, comprises a number of stages from filling the basin and opening the shampoo bottle to drying the hair or cleaning the basin after use. The number of separate performances which the occupational therapist identify in order to teach a task will depend on the individual patient's capacity for learning. Ability to complete the entire task involves chained learning of each stage.

Backward chaining is the strategy of teaching the final stage first and working backwards towards completion of the whole task. The main advantage lies in the additional reinforcement gained by the patient in having completed the task on each occasion. For example, in teaching a mentally handicapped child to put his own socks on, the final stage of pulling them up is taught first. The satisfaction which he gains is used to motivate the learning of earlier parts of the task.

Social skills training

Social skills training is the last of the techniques to be described here. Although the methods involved are essentially behavioural, the associated concepts of self-development look forward to the next chapter on humanistic influences.

Social skills training involves the acquisition of effective social behaviours in order to fulfil personal needs. If such skills normally are learnt throughout childhood and adult life then it follows that they may be taught deliberately to those who lack them. The process is one of making a careful assessment or analysis of present social behaviour, setting graded goals and then designing a training programme to achieve these goals.

Analysis of present behaviour should include verbal and non-verbal elements of communication and habitual strategies in communication. Verbal elements include tone of voice, pitch, volume and clarity as well as the actual content of speech. A monotonous voice or a voice which is too quiet or too loud is difficult to listen to. Speech habits which affect the clarity of the content also include talking too quickly or too slowly, clipping or slurring of words or using too many 'ums' and 'ers' as speech fillers. Some people tend to leave sentences unfinished, are repetitious or are over-emphatic. All these common features of speech, when present to excess, affect the individual's ability to communicate.

Non-verbal elements include the use of eye contact, which may be lacking, inappropriate or too intense. Facial expression is equally important: contact is maintained or altered by the interest or reactions expressed facially by participants in conversation. Physical proximity and orientation are significant in establishing the degree of intimacy which exists between two people. Discomfort or misunderstanding can arise when a person places himself physically closer than is appropriate to the relationship or when he distances himself in space. Attitudes conveyed through posture or degree of tension contribute to communication as do gestures and habitual mannerisms.

Not least in the significant elements of non-verbal communication is physical appearance, including style and appropriateness of dress, cleanliness and choices of personal adornment. This is not a complete catalogue of the factors contributing to social interaction but is intended to suggest the extent required of any assessment and subsequent training programme.

Training goals may be devised in relation to specific problems that a patient has or to personal ambitions that he wishes to fulfil. Alternatively a training programme which is pertinent to problems experienced by a number of patients may be designed. In this case individuals are assessed for their suitability to join the training group.

It is important that goals should be carefully graded when used either for individuals or for groups. Social skills are arranged hierarchically according to complexity and to the degree of anxiety which they may provoke. Each skill is acquired and rehearsed before the next is attempted. An example of an early goal is to achieve ease in a casual exchange of greeting. Later goals may involve competence in self-presentation in a formal setting, such as an interview, or developing a relationship desirable to the patient in a social context.

Training sessions follow a regular pattern. A topic is selected, such as use of eye contact, initiating a conversation, giving information or refusing a request. The skills involved are demonstrated by a model, preferably someone with whom the patient can identify. The patient then imitates and modifies the performance through role-play. Feedback, which should be specific and constructive, is given on the effectiveness of the patient's performance. The feedback may involve therapists, other patients or the use of videotape recording. The corrected behaviour is then practised.

'Homework assignments' are used to transfer the training to real-life situations. The patient is expected to apply the skill learnt to a social setting outside the training group, before the next session. At the beginning of each session there is a recapitulation of the skills learnt previously. Each patient reports back on his 'homework', discussing not only the effectiveness of this performance but also the degree of stress experienced in carrying it out.

BIBLIOGRAPHY

Boles R C 1975 Learning theory. Holt, Reinhart and Winston, New York
Butler R A 1953 Discrimination learning by rhesus monkeys to visual exploration. Motivation Journal of Comparitive Psychology 46: 95–98
Harlow H F, Harlow M K, Meyer D R 1950 Learning motivated by a manipulation drive. Journal of Experimental Psychology 40: 228–34
Miller N E 1969 Learning of visceral and glandular responses. Science 163: 434–445
Spence J T, Carson R C, Thibault J W (eds) 1976 Behavioural approaches to therapy. General Learning Press, Morristown, New Jersey
Trower P, Bryant B, Argyle M 1978 Social skills and mental health. Methuen, London
Wolfe J B 1936 Effectiveness of token-rewards for chimpanzees. Comparative Psychology Monographs 12, No 60
Wolpe J 1958 Psychotherapy by reciprocal inhibition. Stanford University Press, California

RECOMMENDED READING

Blackman D 1974 Operant conditioning — an experimental analysis of behaviour. Methuen, London
Borger R, Seaborne A E M 1976 The psychology of learning. Penguin, Harmondsworth
Burns R B 1980 Essential psychology. MTP Press, Lancaster
Cashdan A, Whitehead J (eds) 1971 Personality growth and learning. The Open University Press and Longman, London

Cohen J, Clark J H 1979 Medicine, mind and man. Freeman, Reading
Cotter B S, Guerra J J 1976 Assertion training. Research Press, Illinois
Deibert A N, Harman A J 1970 New tools for changing behaviour. Research
    Press, Illinois
Hebb D O 1949 Organisation of behaviour. Wiley, New York
Hill W F 1972 Learning, 2nd edn. Methuen, London
Jehu D 1967 Learning theory and social work. Routledge and Kegan Paul,
    London
Johnson C W, Snibbe J R, Evans L A 1980 Basic psychotherapeutics: a
    programmed text, MTP Press, Lancaster
Liberman R P, King L W, DeRisi W J, McCann M 1975 Personal
    effectiveness. Research Press, Illinois
Priestley P, McGuire P, Flegg D, Hemsley V, Welham D 1978 Social skills
    and personal problem solving. Tavistock, London
Strongman K T 1979 Psychology for the paramedical professions. Croom
    Helm, London

2

The humanistic influence

The group of patients with whom we are concerned is numerically very large. It can be tempting to think in terms of categories such as the mentally handicapped, the chronic psychotics, the disordered personalities and the elderly mentally infirm. Such categorization is convenient but can lead to a failure to perceive each patient as being unique. Since therapists, students and helpers are convinced of their own unique existence it may be helpful to consider the needs and the development of all people as individuals.

Some patients may have an unusual perception of the world of which they are a part; some therapists may forget that their own needs and self-expression form a part of the environment in which the patient is treated. The views summarized here are relevant not only to the planning of treatment for individual patients but also to the continuing growth and personal development of each therapist.

ROOTS AND BRANCHES

When you start reading about humanistic psychology, or the human potential movement in therapy, there is a rapid confrontation with such words as 'existential', 'phenomenological' or 'experiential'. Fortunately no word is so long that it cannot be cut down to size by the processes of definition.

Existentialism is not a therapy or a technique but an approach to 'being-in-the-world'. It has its roots in oriental and central European philosophy and found its expression in the West particularly in the works of Jean-Paul Sartre and Albert Camus. 'Being-in-the-world' is a phrase which is intended to convey the interdependence of the individual and his environment. I have no existence which is apart from the world in which I live. This world is made up of my physical and thinking self, the people around me and their responses, and the physical environment or landscape. The world as I know it has no existence apart from me; its reality is dependent upon my experiencing it and expressing it.

Because man's environment is essentially his view and expression of it, causes and effects cannot be separated in the stimulus–response explanations of human behaviour adopted by the behaviourists. I do things because I *understand* my world and because in doing them I make it real. To simplify things I shall make another cup of coffee. I shall turn the kettle off when the water boils because I understand that if I do not it will boil dry. In drinking the coffee I express my physical and emotional existence. Me, the kettle, the coffee and the sensation of drinking, are all together in the present tense. We are a transient moment of my reality. Other parts of this fragment of existence are the sound of my neighbour putting out milk bottles, and my own experience of worry that I may not be summarising existentialism coherently.

How then can this idea of existentialism contribute to either explaining human maladjustment or providing philosophies of treatment?

If I am not an object that is controlled by a separate environment, then it follows in existential thinking that I am both free and also responsible for my own existence. This can cause me a few problems. Firstly, I cannot blame my friends, relations or 'situations beyond my control' for my own inadequacies or misfortunes. If I am not the effect of a whole load of causes then the ball stops in my court. Secondly, I can fail to represent myself truly, preferring to be controlled by others or to deny my own potential. The person who denies or 'blocks' his own grounds for existence will tend to become dependent on the expectations of others, experience guilt and depression as a result of failing to fulfil himself, and perhaps become confused about his own separate identity.

Phenomenology is the tool of the existentialist. A phenomenon is simply a thing or piece of information which is perceived. My fears, my coffee drinking, my neighbour's milk bottles and my heartbeat are all phenomena. Phenomenology in the existential sense seeks to understand the psychological phenomena of behaviour. It does not seek to explain them in terms of cause and effect but to bring them to consciousness as part of the perceived present. To experience 'wholeness' as a person it is necessary to recognize and to understand the phenomena which make up individual behaviour in the context of the immediate environment. It is this consciousness which allows the individual to behave authentically as 'being-in-the-world'.

The relationship between the existentialist approach to living and the practice of therapy can be traced to many sources, for example the work of the philosopher Martin Heidegger (1889–1976) or the existential analyst Ludwig Binswanger (1881–1966). The major influence is in the nature of the relationship between the therapist and the patient or client. Instead of an analytical or a controlling relationship there needs to be an active dialogue, with the therapist attempting to share the patient's experience of reality. The therapist, according to Binswanger (1955) 'will not turn the patient into an object in contrast to himself as subject but will regard him as a partner in human reality'.

R. D. Laing (1960) describes his work *The Divided Self* as an 'existential-phenomenological account' and within it he applies these concepts to the problems presented by psychosis. He describes the psychotic patient as having ideas about himself or about reality which are incongruent with the world as experienced by 'sane' people. He may describe himself as being dead, as being made of glass, as disintegrating or as being Christ or Napoleon. Such beliefs may be real to him, in an existential sense. But they cut him off from the shared reality which allows normal people to be accessible to each other through communication and relationship.

Such incongruence has arisen from the patient's social history, particularly in relation to his family. This is different from describing the symptoms of schizophrenia as related to disease in the medical sense. R. D. Laing and his associate David Cooper, who together wrote *Reason and Violence* in 1964, describe their approach as being 'antipsychiatry'. The proposed strategy of the therapist is to attempt to share the patient's experience with him, withdrawing from the custodial roles more often associated with institutional care. Experimental projects involving schizophrenic patients were described by Laing in *The Divided Self* and by Cooper in *Psychiatry and Antipsychiatry* (1967). These projects are no longer running but the philosophies of care propounded by these authors and others have influenced current ideas about treatment and long-term care.

Existentialism has been given space here since it is perhaps the major influence on humanistic psychology. The other roots are numerous and include neo-Freudian and Jungian philosophies as well as an integration of modern American ideology. The simplest way of approaching it is to say that it centres on the potential of man. A humanistic attitude is based on the idea that man can improve himself by his own efforts.

To give a bit more substance to these ideas this chapter will go on to examine briefly the work of Carl Rogers and Abraham Maslow, both of whom belong to the humanistic school of psychology and have had considerable influence on the present-day practice of therapy.

CARL ROGERS

The concept of self

Central to an understanding of the contribution of Carl Rogers to humanist psychology is an appreciation of his use of the term 'self'. Unfortunately this word has been given slightly different meanings by a number of different theorists so it is easy to become confused about what is being implied by its use. It can mean the total of all that a person feels about himself, the way in which he thinks, perceives others and responds to his environment. This is obviously a very broad definition. Some, on the other hand, prefer to limit the term 'self' to an individual's concept of his own being, a personal identity rather than an inclusion of all psychological processes and actions. The definition and relevence to occupational therapy of theories of self will be given a bit more space in Chapter 3.

Carl Rogers is concerned with self-concept, a series of beliefs or a view of oneself which may be partly conscious and partly unconscious. The self- concept which an individual has will affect the way in which he experiences, perceives and responds to events. For example, two girls whistled at in the street will experience that event differently and impute to it different meanings. One may feel flattered, amused and inclined to respond. The other may be embarrassed, irritated or even alarmed. The whistle is the same but the self-concept of each of the girls is different and will mediate the experience, its meaning and the response.

Rogers describes the individual as tending to develop in ways which are consistent with his existing structure of self-concepts. Thus a person who believes himself to be less intelligent or more clumsy than others will not elect to invest too much in activities which depend on these attributes for success. Believing oneself to be generous or good-natured leads to a development of these qualities. The important thing is that a well-adjusted individual should be able to express the self that he conceives himself to be, in words or actions.

A congruence between the individual's total experience of and participation in his environment and his accurate awareness of self makes him a *fully functioning person*. Lack of such congruence can be seen in an example of someone behaving in a way which does not agree with his structure of self-concepts. You may think of yourself as being particularly patient in your associations with elderly infirm people who are, perhaps, slow or confused. The day that you snap irritably at one of these under your care, your resulting feeling of unease or dismay may well find expression in such phrases as 'I wasn't myself' or 'I don't know what came over me'. The behaviour has to be disowned in order to preserve the self-concept.

If this simple example is extended, it is possible to appreciate the discomfort of a person who consistently fails to represent himself as the self that he believes himself to be. The lack of congruence becomes a gap between an ideal self and an actual self. If this is the case, general dissatisfaction and disturbance is a likely outcome.

The process of expressing and developing the self is one of self-actualization. The ability to self-actualize varies between individuals, but in Rogerian theory this is seen to be a major motivating force and goal in life.

Rogerian therapy

Self-actualization is important to the individual. Lack of congruity between experience and self-concept leads to maladjustment. The maladjusted individual cannot actualize his potential since he will frequently reject feelings and actions which are not consistent with his self-image. Rogers therefore suggests that a healthy individual is able to change or adapt the self in order to maintain congruity with a changing environment.

Take, for example a person whose self-concept is of a shy and passive individual but whose survival or happiness within his social context requires a more forceful or demanding approach. He must either adapt his perceived self in order that it should allow him to operate effectively or he must fall back on unrewarding attempts merely to defend an unsatisfactory self-concept.

It has already been said that a humanistic view claims the ability of man to understand himself and to change or improve through his own efforts. The techniques of Rogerian therapy are directed towards helping the patient, or client, to make the necessary changes in his own life and especially in his own structure of self-concepts.

The method proposed is known as non-directive or client-centred therapy. His basic philosophy is that change can be facilitated by a therapist entering into a warm and supportive relationship with the client in which an *unconditional positive regard* is shown for the client whatever he says or does. If the client feels respected and valued by another person this allows him to express his less desirable feelings or behaviours, knowing that they will be accepted. In doing this he may gain enough support and confidence to examine and accept the more negative aspects of himself or his experience instead of relying on defence mechanisms.

The major technique involved is that of reflecting back to the client his own speech or actions whilst communicating total acceptance. It is important not simply to reflect, as a mirror would, any statement that the client makes but to demonstrate a genuine empathy and regard for him as a person.

This form of therapy has been applied to a wide range of human problems. It can be used within play therapy with children and has been developed particularly to help those experiencing periods of stress related to adolescence or to adult relationships.

The long-term psychiatric patient has special problems of maintaining self-esteem. His concept of self will be affected not only by any condition which he may have been diagnosed as having but also by his situation as a dependent patient within an institution. Rogers & Dymond (1954) used these principles in the treatment of patients within psychiatric hospitals and their results, supported by other subsequent studies, found them to be at least partially effective. Self-esteem increases when there is greater congruence between the self and ideal self. Patients showing these changes also improved according to other criteria of recovery.

In the application of client-centred therapy to hospitalized schizophrenics the success of treatment was found to relate to the therapist's own ability to define himself and be aware of the dynamics of the interaction of himself and the patient (Rogers et al, 1967). This seems to confirm that congruence within the therapist's own personality becomes an important influence on the effectiveness of his work with patients.

The demand that a client-centred approach makes on both therapist and patient are not, however, all that profound. It does not call for deeply analytical or interpretative ability which, in the case of the psychotic patient, may not be present. What is required is an ability to communicate well and to form an appropriate relationship with the client. This may not be easy since empathy and unconditional positive regard must be genuinely felt and not merely contrived or pretended as part of a technical performance.

ABRAHAM MASLOW

The name of Maslow is associated with the hierarchy of needs that he suggests as a basis for human motivation, and with self-actualization. Although it is a pity not to discuss his work and that of Carl Rogers more broadly, a basic review of theory here must be limited to these two topics.

Hierarchy of human needs

All animals, including man, are driven to act in order to satisfy their own needs. The sophistication of these needs differs according to the potential or the complexity of the animal. Mankind regards himself as the most complex of all animals.

Maslow arranges human needs in a hierarchical order. The more basic needs have to be at least partially satisfied as a prerequisite to striving to fulfil higher needs. A sequence of categories of needs is used.

Physiological needs

These are for the essential things like food, water and oxygen. They relate to the primary reinforcers discussed in the previous chapter as being essential to life. To most people these only become important when they are absent, in which case everything else loses significance until these basic requirements are assured once more.

Safety needs

In order to explore, experience and develop, the individual needs to know a measure of security. Activity, other than avoidance, is discouraged by a feeling of impending danger. Safety is a straightforward need if you relate it to physical hazards, such as sitting on top of a volcano or being blown up by a bomb.

However, a feeling of safety is not simply the absence of any obvious threat. To feel safe with other people and within the social and physical environment it is necessary to understand and to be able to predict everyday events. It is necessary to be a part of society, sharing reality with others and reaching a common appreciation of both an ordered and a changing world. Because we need to be safe we explore and seek to understand the world in which we live. It is a contemporary problem that, even when an individual has achieved a feeling of being safe within his own social group and immediate surroundings, his environment may still be threatened by world events such as the possibility of nuclear war. So this is not just a straightforward need, to be resolved as hunger is by a hot dinner. The world in which we live has constructed and maintains its own basic anxieties.

Needs for love and belonging

Once the two previous concerns have been resolved as far as possible, the individual needs to feel that he is loved and accepted for himself. To feel worthy of love involves more than just doing things that other people approve of; it requires that one is valued for being oneself.

Think back to Carl Roger's unconditional positive regard: the client-centred therapist is surely attempting to fulfil the client's need for love and belonging by accepting him for himself. Fulfilment of this need allows a self-concept which is both positive and optimistic. The institutionalized patient is likely to have difficulty in forming such a self-concept since, although he may receive affection from staff or others, this is often conditional on him behaving in certain ways or meeting expectations based on his role as a patient.

Esteem needs

It is one thing to be loved and accepted for oneself alone, but then comes an additional need to achieve something, to gain respect or recognition as a productive and able person. Most people at some time long to excel at one thing. Even if there are no competitive ambitions involved, in terms of being better than average, no-one really enjoys having a lesser status or being seen as less productive or less meaningful.

Here again the style of life experienced by long-term psychiatric patients can produce examples of difficulties in fulfilling this need. When work activities or industrial rehabilitation are discussed later in this book it will inevitably mean referring back to the need for esteem or status as a major reason for using this form of treatment. It must be remembered, however, that recognition is not only gained by working at a task effectively. Status is also given to those who successfully perform within distinct roles, for example as parent, counsellor, entertainer, helper, sportsman or intellectual.

Cognitive and aesthetic needs

These are concerned with a satisfying relationship between the individual and his culture. Knowing and exploring the physical and social world can also involve an appreciation of order, natural form and beauty. Exploration need not take the form of paddling up the Amazon in a canoe. Interest in the ideas of another person, experiences involving music and the visual arts, opportunities to gain knowledge or to learn new skills are all forms of exploration. The greatest 'explorers' personally known to you are likely to be involved people who are concurrently concerned with the successfull fulfilment of all the other needs already discussed.

Self-actualization

The idea of 'self-actualization' has already been mentioned. Rogers, in using this term, gives it a meaning similar to his 'fully functioning person'. Literally it means making one's self real. The expression of self is associated with the development of knowledge about oneself and with the acceptance of the relationship between self and the environment.

Maslow (1954) defines abnormality as 'Anything that frustrates or blocks or denies the essential nature of man' and psychopathological as 'Anything that disturbs or frustrates or twists the course of self-actualization'. It naturally follows that therapy of any kind should be motivated towards enabling the individual to reach a position from which self-actualization becomes a possibility.

If self-actualization is the goal of the healthy individual, how does this relate to the treatment of long-term psychiatric patients who are unable to fulfil more basic needs? The inclusion of self-actualization here is intended to provide a perspective on both the level of difficulties that a patient is experiencing and the level of function that he may attain. It has also been suggested that fully congruent therapists may be more effective in forming relationships with patients. Congruent therapists in this context maybe identified by their ability to actualize themselves, and in so doing increase and accept awareness of themselves and the way in which they work. This second point has a significance, to members of any caring profession, in terms of a responsibility towards self-development and the personal development of staff.

Maslow developed the concept of self-actualization by studing apparently successful and well-adjusted personalities rather than studying the disturbed or the neurotic. Thus his view of man is essentially optimistic and emphasises the natural disposition of each individual to make full use of his own abilities.

Maslow recognizes that a number of self-actualizing personalities have features in common. These features include spontaneity, realism, independence and an appreciation of other people, problem-solving ability, privacy and a non-destructive sense of humour. They resist stereotyping and are capable of deep and accepting relationships. He also describes self-actualizers as having 'peak experiences of extreme pleasure, which may derive from real events but involve feelings beyond time and place'. It cannot be easy to be a consistent self-actualizer and it is somewhat discouraging to have Einstein, Beethoven and Eleanor Roosevelt quoted as examples of people who, in Maslow's view, actually achieved this. It is quite a goal, though, to reach beyond or 'transcend' the constrictions of self-concept.

Towards the end of his life, Maslow (1973) suggested two categories of people who were able to meet the basic hierarchical needs and were thus able to attempt fulfilment of full human potential. The first group he describes as the 'merely healthy' and the other group as 'transcenders'. There is nothing wrong with being merely healthy and such individuals are strong personalities with clear views of their own strengths and weaknesses and well-defined personal objectives. They are happy, efficient and effective. In working with patients we aim to reinstate health. A transcender is stirred by emotional peaks of experience, profound relationships and the resolution of moral and philosophical dichotomies, together with a clear knowledge of his own fluid self-concept.

This has perhaps gone far enough to indicate that discussion of humanistic influences can quickly give rise to question about the way in which we live, the values we hold and the decisions we make. These factors affect not only the management of our own lives but also those of patients whose situation makes them vulnerable to the attitudes of those who 'care' for them.

HUMANISTIC INFLUENCES AND OCCUPATIONAL THERAPY

A number of different therapeutic methods have arisen from humanistic thought. Client-centred therapy has already been mentioned within the section on Carl Rogers. Gestalt therapy is largely based on humanistic principles although it also has roots in Gestalt psychology and in psychoanalysis.

In Europe, the 'biofunctional therapies' of Wilhelm Reich and, in America, the 'primal therapy' described by Arthur Janov are examples of therapies which are indebted to modern humanistic psychology. The expressive therapies, of particular interest to occupational therapists, such as Moreno's 'psychodrama' share this same base.

These methods or 'therapies' have their major application in the treatment of neurotic disorders and of crises in life. So what is this chapter doing in a book devoted to the treatment of long-term psychiatric disorders? The important thing to realize is that the humanistic influence is not simply a source of relatively new methods of treatment but has had an impact on the way in which we view psychiatric illness and the attitudes which we bring to bear on our relationships with patients.

Occupational therapy can be recognised as having a traditionally humanistic base since, like several other caring professions, some of what we do is based on the following ideals:

1. Optimism

Humanistic and existential ideas about man are essentially

optimistic. Unhappiness, abnormality or evil are thought to be due to a failure in fulfilling potential rather than to be an intrinsic tendency. There are positive rewards of joy and a feeling of well-being to be gained by actualizing one's own potential and being able to meet one's own needs.

An occupational therapist does not only seek to identify problems but to help an individual to reach his own potential. Therapy is not directed towards manipulating the patient into doing what someone else thinks he should do; instead, he is encouraged to identify his own preferred goals and to find ways of expressing his own personality. The therapist tries to motivate and to encourage him by believing in his capacity for self-improvement and by being both accepting and optimistic about him as an individual.

2. Opportunity

Some disciplines do things to patients in order to assist their recovery and others hope that, given opportunity, patients will do things for themselves. Occupational therapists normally belong to the second category. This means that the occupational therapist is particularly interested in the patient's ability to make choices and to express preferences. The patient who is engaged in purposeful activity of his own choice may be seen to have progressed further than the patient who is engaged in a task specified by the therapist. If a person can achieve independence not only in carrying out tasks but also in determining what he wants to do then he is likely to perceive himself as being a more worthwhile individual.

The occupational therapy department attempts to provide a range of opportunities for the patient to direct his own activity, and to experiment in playing roles other than those of dependency and passivity which are often associated with his status as a patient.

3. Emphasis on the 'whole person'

First year occupational therapy students often state that they have been attracted to the profession because it perceives the patient as a whole rather than restricts treatment to the part which seems to have gone wrong. This is a considerable claim, but at least it illustrates the first concern, that of optimism.

There is an undeniable stress on the connection between physical and mental health. Physical exercise, sport and relaxation are encouraged because an improvement in the psychiatric patient's physical health is seen to have an impact on his mood and self-concept. Emphasis is placed on the patient's physical appearance and decisions that he is able to make about personal hygiene, dress and grooming. Personal awareness and individuality of appearance are recognized as important to the recovery of a patient who is presented as being depressed, apathetic or lacking in self-confidence. The occupational therapist is also concerned with diet — a hot dinner may not cure all psychological ills but it is part of the total picture. A concern for physical health and appearance and for a balanced diet contributes towards a patient's perception of himself as a healthy and valuable individual able to progress to the fulfilment of higher needs.

4. Focus on individual needs

Maslow's hierarchy of needs and his reference to humanistic psychology as a 'third force', the other two being behaviourism and psychoanalysis, have had a considerable impact on occupational therapy. The profession has traditionally rated personal growth as high, if not higher, than the reduction of symptoms. The assessment of a patient is not limited to recording what is wrong with him and what things he cannot do. It is equally important to know what he can do, what he would like to do and what limitations are being placed on his ability to meet his own needs as an individual.

Take an example from physical rehabilitation for a change. Only the most unimaginative therapist will devote hours to insisting that a hemiplegic patient should learn to peel potatoes with one hand when his greatest personal need is to maintain specific social relationships. He is better off eating instant potato and gaining sufficient confidence and energy to get down to the pub.

5. Emphasis on interpersonal relationship

An occupational therapist is likely to resist being described as simply a director of activity. The relationship and the dialogue between therapist and patient are given equal importance with the performance of practical skills. There are two important factors to be considered: the quality of communication with the patient and the personal development or maturity of the therapist. It is sometimes stated that the first task of the occupational therapist is to form a 'rapport' with the patient. This sounds splendid but also, perhaps, a little vague. Manford H. Kuhn (1961) discussing professional relationships gives an interesting, if complex, definition:

> Rapport is probably by no means the intangible, mysterious thing it has been characterised as being. It involves, at bottom, simply the sharing of a common language, so that through shared frames of reference each person in what he has to say, or in each posture he takes, calls out in himself, incipiently, the response that these gestures, postures and symbols call out in the other.

The frame of reference being used by Kuhn is that of symbolic interaction, and rather than translate his statement for those unfamiliar with this frame, the discussion of interpersonal relationships will be the central theme of the next chapter. This will seek to explain the basic concepts of symbolic interactionism and to use these to discuss the interaction between the patient and the therapist.

BIBLIOGRAPHY

Binswanger L 1955 Ausgewahlte Vortrage and Aufsatze Vol 2 quoted in Kovel, op cit.
Cooper D G 1967 Psychiatry and antipsychiatry, Tavistock, London
Hall S H, Lindzey G 1970 Theories of personality, 2nd edn. John Wiley, New York
Harper R A 1975 The new psychotherapies. Prentice-Hall Englewood Cliffs, New Jersey
Kovel J 1976 A complete guide to therapy. Penguin, Harmondsworth
Kuhn M H 1962 The interview and the professional relationship. In: Rose A M (ed) Human behaviour and social processes Routledge and Kegan Paul, London
Laing R D 1960, The divided self. Tavistock, London

Laing R D, Cooper D G 1964 Reason and violence. Penguin,
    Harmondsworth
Maslow A H 1973 The farther reaches of human nature. Penguin,
    Harmondsworth
Rogers C R (ed) 1967 The therapeutic relationship and its impact: a study
    of psychotherapy with schizophrenics. University of Wisconsin Press,
    Madison, Wisconsin
Rogers C R 1967 On becoming a person. Constable, London
Rogers C R, Dymond R F 1954 (eds) Psychotherapy and personality change,
    co-ordinated studies in the clients centred approach. University of
    Chicago Press, Chicago

RECOMMENDED READING

Carkhuff R R, Berenson B G 1967 Beyond counseling and therapy, 2nd edn.
    Holt, Rinehart and Winston, New York
Coulter J 1973 Approaches to insanity. Martin Robertson, London
Fidler G S, Fidler J W 1978 Doing and becoming: purposeful action and
    self-actualization. American Journal of Occupational Therapy 32:5,
    305–310
Hindess B 1977 Philosophy and methodology in the social sciences. The
    Harvester Press, Hassocks, Sussex
Perls F S, Hefferline R F, Goodman G 1951 Gestalt therapy. Penguin,
    Harmondsworth
Rowan J 1983 The reality game. Routledge and Kegan Paul, London

3

Self, socialization and occupational therapy

Theories underlying occupational therapy draw from a wide range of disciplines. Theories of learning, for example, have been contributed mainly by psychologists. Theories of self, developing from humanistic ideas discussed in the previous chapter, arise from the borders of social psychology and sociology.

It is not possible, or not wise, to consider a patient in isolation from his social context. His interaction with others, which includes the way in which they view him, is an important part of his identity. Occupational therapy utilize social environments and its practice, therefore, must be based on a knowledge of social relationships.

SYMBOLIC INTERACTION

'Symbolic interaction' is concerned with the meanings that we attach to our own and to other people's intentions and actions. Interactionist theory arises from the work of a number of sociologists and social psychologists. Unlike the mainstream of sociology which examines organizations and relationships on a large scale, symbolic interactionists are interested in small scale social interactions such as individual social encounters. Unlike the mainstream of psychology which examines the minutiae of behaviour in all vertebrates, including man, social interactionists are specifically concerned with communication between people and the social meanings that these may involve.

The 'symbolic' half of symbolic interaction represents an interest in your use of symbols to convey meaning. A symbol is anything that a number of people agree to use in order to communicate a meaning or a value. A red light is a symbol of danger, by common agreement. Words are symbols: the word 'table' means something flat which is raised off the ground and upon which other things may be placed. The word 'like' does not have such obvious meaning in the visual or tactile sense but carries certain values. The thumbs up sign is a symbol which transcends language, and so is a smile. This all seems rather obvious until one tries to visualize a social world which is without symbols which can be learned and applied to create mutual understanding. Human interaction would grind to a standstill, or at least be exceedingly chaotic.

Some symbols acquire particular meanings within specific social groups, for instance 'the book' has different usage for a group of evangelical missionaries and a group of Football Association referees. Because the meaning of symbols can be socially defined in this way there is plenty of room for misunderstanding: to 'knock someone up' has a different meaning either side of the Atlantic.

Members of caring professions frequently use words such as 'socialization', 'self' and 'role' in describing either patients or the intentions of treatment. Part of the purpose of including this chapter is to examine whether we do all mean the same thing when these terms are used, and to further mutual understanding of these concepts.

Apart from making factual exchanges possible, the use of symbols has several important functions. One of these is to enable an individual to 'take the role of another'. To 'take the role of another' is to empathize with him, or to experience a situation from his point of view. Applying the same meaning to symbols allows one person to imagine how another might feel about or understand a situation and to predict what his response might be. The simplest example is when someone winces when he sees another crack his head on a low beam.

Role taking is, however, central to communication since the communicator constructs his message by imagining how the recipient might understand it. Only because it is possible to emphathize with another is it possible to influence his behaviour.

If, for example, you are a student, then you may have no difficulty in empathizing with another student of similar age and background who is following the same course of study. In your communication it is possible to evoke in yourself the way in which the other understands that communication. That is fine, but there is more than one other person in the world. Not only can one take the role of another but one can also 'generalize' to evoke simultaneously the responses of a whole social group of people. In this way one can not only communicate within a particular society but also actively belong within it.

A culture is an elaborate set of meanings and values which is learnt and accepted by each of its members and is communicated both by the use of symbols and by the ability of each member to predict the understanding and responses of the others. The word 'culture' can be applied very broadly or can be used to describe a specialized subgroup within society. Sharing a culture enables people to have certain expectations of each other's behaviour based on common meanings and values. This is one of the main features of a society as opposed to a collection of individuals.

What is the significance of this? We all operate as members of society without wishing to be confused by a whole structure of sociological jargon. It becomes more interesting when one considers what happens when such features of society are not present. Sommer & Osmond (1962) argued that groups of long-term patients living together on wards of psychiatric hospitals constitute neither societies, cultures nor communities. This argument is based on a typical absence of organization between patients, of reciprocated friendship, and even of conversation.

This may seem a fairly extreme view, particularly since recent years have seen a greater emphasis on social activity within psychiatric hospitals. Such activity is however initiated by staff and does not always redress the lack of social structure and leadership amongst the patients themselves. In the context of schizophrenia, Ernest Becker (1968) also recognizes these problems. He relates the condition to faulty socialization which results in inadequate performance of the social rituals characterizing any given culture.

There is an obvious circular argument arising from the relationship between mental illness and inadequate social performance. Does mental illness arise from social inadequacy or does it give rise to such inadequacy as a result of the environments in which patients live or are treated? This is a question which is central to many problems of diagnosis and care of patients but to which there is no answer applicable to every individual situation. The study of social learning and social behaviour is, however, necessary if social activities are to be used as a form of treatment. The next sections will therefore examine briefly the relationship between socialization and self-concept and the significance of both social role and career.

SELF-CONCEPT AND SOCIALIZATION

In the view of G. H. Mead (1934), a leading figure within interactionist theory, the 'self' arises out of social experience. This self is a constantly changing structure because it is made up of beliefs and attitudes that a person holds about himself, and because these beliefs and attitudes are influenced by the responses of other people around him. In order to view himself objectively he needs to be able to see himself through the eyes of other people. This is a different facet of the role-taking or empathetic ability already discussed.

If you hold certain opinions about yourself, that you are kindly, intelligent, cowardly, or that your nose is too big, these opinions are either altered or verified by other people that you are in contact with. Expressing yourself as you believe yourself to be is a way of asking for and gaining information from others which either validates or modifies the perceptions of self currently held. These responses from other people are, of course, translated. It is what we think people mean which is significant, not what they intend to convey. Sometimes perception may be sufficiently accurate for these two meanings, the conveyed and the received, to be the same, but there is as often a discrepancy.

Identity, in the eyes of others and in the personal view of self, is not confined to having qualities or features such as those used in the above example. Who you are is deeply influenced by the society to which you belong, the roles that you play, your status in relation to other people and the knowledge or abilities that you are recognized as having. These factors are continually changing, which is another reason for describing the self as being essentially fluid.

All this tends to suggest that the identity of any individual is simply a combined reflection of the ways in which other people see him. This can be illustrated by the example of bereavement. When someone of personal importance dies, you miss both that person as an individual and also the unique way in which he or she perceived you. A part of your self has also died. Too simple? If you can convince me that you have a spiritual being or identity which is quite separate from social causes or the views of other people then my view of you may be of someone who is skilled in philosophical argument or who is directed by religious faith. Accept this estimation of you and integrate it into your view of self and you are at least half way to losing the argument.

Fortunately religion, like politics, is beyond the scope of this book. What is important, though, is whether views held about a patient by those concerned with his care contribute to the way in which a patient views himself.

Primary socialization

Socialization is the continuing process through which the self is developed and modified. it may be divided into primary and secondary phases.

Primary socialization occurs in early childhood and is centred on the family. An individual is not born into the world with a ready-made concept of self and recognition of others. He has to go through the process of making the world his own by gradually coming to understand and to participate in its social meanings and language. He learns to identify with those immediate to him and to adopt their interpretation of situations and of symbols. These immediate people, normally the family or small social group into which the child is born, are known as the 'significant others'.

A baby does not choose his significant others, or the race, creed, attitudes and social perceptions which contribute to his early view of objective reality. These significant others control the individual's primary socialization first by acting as a sieve and second by acting as a pair of tinted spectacles. The sieving is the selection of experience and opportunity, often determined by the social class or geographical location. Contrast, for example, the child of the farm labourer with the child of the city-dwelling business man. The tinted spectacles represent the attitudes or opinions which are prevalent. It is quite likely that two children may be born into families of similar class, environment or opportunity but for one to be imbued with a sense of contentment and the other with bitter resentment.

So, primary socialization gives each individual a springboard; he belongs within a small part of society and can take the role of significant others in determining his own 'self-concept' and behaviour. He has learnt role taking through being controlled and also through play. What child doesn't act out roles of mother, father, head of state or imaginary friend in fantasy and in experiment?

Because primary socialization is dependent on the chance of birth, then when it is unsatisfactory this is also the result of biographical accident. Physical deformities and mental handicap could be described as biological biographical accidents. Extreme poverty, illegitimacy or simply being unwanted are, to the child, accidents of social biography. Such accidents do not inevitably have an unsuccessful result in terms of socialization, but they can, if they carry social stigma, affect the concept of self being formed at this stage. Berger & Luckman (1966) describe the consequences to the individual of bearing such a stigma.

> He *is* what he is supposed to be, to himself as to his significant others and to the community as a whole. To be sure, he may react to this fate with resentment or rage, but it is *qua* inferior being that he is resentful and enraged. His resentment and rage may even serve as decisive ratifications of his socially defined identity as an inferior being, since his betters, by definition, are above these brutish emotions. . . . The unsuc-

cessfully socialized individual himself is socially predefined as a profiled type — the cripple, the bastard, the idiot, and so on.

Secondary socialization

Once a child has established a social life of his own, through school, interests and associations with his peer group, he is subject to a wider range of influences than those provided by the significant others of his primary socialization. This is the point from which *secondary socialization* starts and continues throughout life.

It is no longer enough to take the role of specific individuals in order to determine the behaviour and the identity of the self. This would place severe limitations on individual growth and development. Instead, there is a move towards generalization, the individual adopts attitudes towards social activities or undertakings common to the society, or groups within the society, to which he belongs. The people whose view of reality is important to him become a much larger group and are known as the 'generalized other'. In perceiving himself, and in other forms of thought, the individual now takes the attitude of the generalized other toward himself. Being a member of a social group in this way exerts a control on the individual.

If you are not quite clear what is meant by being controlled by the attitudes and norms of behaviour which a social group brings to bear on its individual members, then try a simple experiment. List the reasons, other than financial, which inhibit you from boarding a bus tomorrow morning and presenting a banana to each of your fellow passengers.

Secondary socialization normally arises from membership of more than one social group. One person may belong simultaneously to a profession, a political party, a sporting association and an informal group of friends. His membership of each has been obtained in different ways. For example, joining a profession involves going through some formal process of acquiring knowledge and becoming accepted by fellow professionals. Joining a political party involves adopting a whole structure of opinion or attitudes. There are many other groups which are less organized or less dependent on social contacts, for example, groups of elderly isolated people, music lovers, gamblers and home brewing enthusiasts. In order to examine why an individual identifies himself as belonging to particular groups and how other people make his claims legitimate, the terms 'role', 'status' and 'career' are used.

Role, status and career

It has already been stated that role-taking is central to symbolic interactionism. Being able to imagine how the other perceives a communication allows that communication to go on. But an individual may have a number of different *roles*, each one adopted according to his relationship with the other actors within a situation. One minute he may be father to his son, and the next, subservient employee, supervisor, dissatisfied customer, illicit lover, expert golfer and casual friend.

When two people meet they quickly reach a consensus as to their relative roles. Sometimes this is straightforward: one often hears said of another person 'you know where you are with him'. Actually it would be more precise to say you know *who* you are, the relative roles are well defined and the expectations of each other are clear. Sometimes it is not so easy: problems may arise from the other person having several possible alternative roles, each of which could be appropriate. For example, the same person may be a friend, a bank manager and a sporting rival. The situation in which he is encountered will be the major influence on the role he assumes or is called upon to play. Quite often the result may be a compromise. If an individual is unhappy about borrowing money from a friend he may be wishing to avoid including the roles of debtor and creditor within the relationship.

It is difficult to discuss roles without also discussing status. A *status* is a collection of duties and rights. Parents, for example, are expected to meet the various needs of their own children but are privileged to make decisions or plans on their behalf until they reach a status which includes the right to determine their own future. A role is a combination of strategies and attitudes used to maintain a status. The role of the teacher in the classroom is a familiar example: what he is and what he does is a performance which is part of having a status as a teacher. His being a teacher may involve other roles in relation to his position within an educational hierarchy, to his friends or to his family.

A status which is reflected by a number of different associated roles is said to have a particular 'role set'. The role set associated with being an occupational therapist may be a combination of the roles adopted in relating to patients, other senior and junior members of the profession, colleagues in other professions and administrators.

Just as the normal person expects to exercise a number of roles he also experiences changes in status. A series of changes in status make up a *career*. This can mean a career in the employment sense but the term can be employed much more broadly. A school or college career involves changes in status with age, examination success and evolving interests. A different type of career may involve courtship, engagement and marriage, with subsequent stages of separation and divorce or a happier and more lasting outcome.

At any one time an individual may be engaged in several different careers, each one involving a different series of changes in status and each status requiring the performance of different roles. Movement from one status to another is known as a 'status passage' which may be accompanied by social rituals such as the marriage ceremony, presentation ceremonies or public announcements. Life does not necessarily go on getting better and better; changes in status may involve sideways or downward moves. Bankruptcy, demotion, retirement, admission to institutional care, childbirth and moving house may all be regarded as status passages which may, or may not, be anticipated with pleasure.

This raises the subject of labelling. Whether one is a student, an occupational therapist, a patient or a teacher it is difficult to avoid being given a label by others. A label carries with it expectations of behaviour, and once labelled there is a tendency to fulfil these expectations. When labels are given which imply positive expectations of wisdom, skill or understanding then the response in terms of behaviour and enhanced self-concept may also be positive. Many labels, however, are applied as a result of social deviance. An ex-convict bears a social label which may frustrate his attempts to earn an honest living. A psychiatric patient may bear two types of label, one being specific such as a diagnosis and the other being the general one of being unable to cope in normal society.

It is very difficult to repudiate a label once applied. Being labelled 'deviant' places oneself outside the accepted norms of society. In response one can either seek professional help or seek the company of others who have been similarly labelled as deviant. Personal relief may result from either of these measures but they also result in the constant reapplication of the label. If occupational therapy is concerned with the re-entry into society of those bearing any physical or psychological stigma then the dynamics of social labelling should be a central concern of its practitioners.

Unfortunately, by simply being employed to offer help to disadvantaged people we are active in the process of labelling them. There is a conscious effort to avoid such terms as 'geriatric', 'subnormal' and, less frequently, 'schizophrenic', but expectations of patients based on their deviant status inevitably affect their self-concept as people.

Self-concept is where all this started and a number of influencing factors have now been identified. The self is a changing structure arising out of social experience. It is influenced by the way in which one perceives others to view oneself. The perceptions of others will be influenced by status, role performance and social labelling amongst other things. The self-concept of a long-term psychiatric patient is likely to include ideas and beliefs which do not make him feel good. These ideas and beliefs may stem from the way in which he is regarded by those responsible for his treatment. Bring to mind any individual patient and try answering this small selection of questions:

— Does he need to be in hospital?
— Do decisions have to be made by others on his behalf?
— If he loses his temper how is this construed?
— Do you enjoy his company enough to want more of it?
— What roles are associated with his status as a psychiatric patient?
— What other roles does he have the opportunity to perform?

ERVING GOFFMAN

Within this section of the book it has been the practice to select and briefly summarize aspects of the work of one or two central contributors to the theme of each chapter. Although there is a wide range of individuals whose work would be valuable in reinforcing the basic concepts of this chapter, the writings of Erving Goffman are particularly tempting since he has applied the concepts of symbolic inter-action to the problems of both physical and psychological abnormality. Two of Goffman's descriptions of the relation-ship between the 'carers' and the 'cared for' illustrate his work. These are the distinction between 'the own and the wise' and the factors determining the 'moral career of the mental patient'.

The own and the wise

The social status of an individual is surmised on a first meeting and subsequently revised or reinforced during subsequent interaction. The impression gained of another person is influenced by his personal appearance, mode of dress, speech, vocabulary, reputation and a number of other visible and less visible clues. A stigma is anything which is different about a person if this affects his acceptability in normal social interaction. Physical abnormalities form one example, but others can include a history of mental illness, criminality, addiction, sexual deviation or even higher intel-lectual ability if this is not a norm within a particular social group.

Goffman (1963) discusses the social response of 'normal' people to those who are discredited by being stigmatized in some way. He says:

> We use specific stigma terms such as cripple, bastard, moron in our daily discourse as a source of metaphor and imagery, typically without giving thought to the original meaning. We tend to impute a wide range of imperfections on the basis of the original one, and at the same time to impute some desir-able but undesired attributes, often of a supernatural cast, such as 'sixth sense', or 'understanding'.

The stigmatized individual comes to recognize himself as being not only different but ashamed or defiled by his differences. If, within his social experiences, he fails to be accepted and respected, then his own view of himself may well concur and He may see his own attributes as deserving such a response. As a response to his own unacceptability the stigmatized person may go to great lengths to find a 'cure' or pursue any course which may serve to ameliorate his shortcomings. he is particularly vulnerable to the advertisement of new forms of therapy, of new methods of achieving intellectual or physical prowess and of possibly fraudulent promises of all kinds. He may well see all the problems experienced within his life as being directly related to the bearing of a stigma, rather than recognizing that 'normal' people may experience equal, if not similar, difficulties.

An individual who has a stigma, whether it takes the form of a physical abnormality or some other deviation, is not alone. Goffman differentiates, between two different groups who are able to offer understanding and support. The first group he terms 'the own'. The own are those who share the same stigma — other people who are equally one-legged, schizophrenic, sensorily impaired, homosexual or whatever. They may meet together as formal associations based on common problems or they may be an informal and mutually recognizing subgroup within society. Certain members of the group of the own may emerge as spokesmen for the group by virtue of being particularly articulate and holding strong views about the necessity to represent publicly the interests of the group. Action groups may be spearheaded by such a 'native' of the group who presents the case on behalf of his stigmatized colleagues. It is possible that, in representing the stigmatized group in such a way, he gains such eminence or recognition within the unstigmatized world that he is no longer truly typical of the group. As Goffman puts it:

> Instead of leaning on their crutch, they get to play golf with it, ceasing, in terms of social participation, to be representative of the people they represent.

The second group are 'the wise'. These are people who are sufficiently close to and concerned with the stigmatized that they carry a sort of courtesy stigma themselves. They may be members of a family with a disabled member or may work closely with the disabled.

The wise accept a stigmatized individual for himself, they require no admission of shame or self-concealment. An individual cannot choose or announce himself to be 'wise'. This status is inferred by the stigmatized or disabled group itself by accepting the outsider as an honorary member of the group. An occupational therapist may be wise in this sense but only as a result of personal re-evaluation and of acceptance by the group of patients served. It may not always be comfortable to be wise; when working within psychiatry or mental handicap the courtesy stigma thus carried may affect other aspects of one's social life. The wise may also potentially embarrass those whom they serve by over-zealous statement of their case or by an overstated moral intensity.

It may seem to be contradictory to be urging moderation at the same time as urging a greater depth of thought in the management of long-term psychiatric patients, but how often are such patients genuinely helped or made to feel accepted by a therapist whose energies are all directed towards the dramatic conversion of the rest of society?

The moral career

The use of the term 'career' has already been discussed; successive changes in work and social status is a common feature of most lives. The moral career described by Goffman (1961) is concerned with a sequence of changes in a person's beliefs about himself and about other people in relation to himself. He is specifically interested in this type of moral career as it occurs in the experiences of psychiatric patients within institutions. These experiences tend to include feelings of being mortified, even though this may not be intended by the staff of the institution.

The majority of residential institutions share certain features with each other. Whereas it is normal to work, sleep and play in different environments and in different company, life in an institution tends to break such barriers down. For example, a patient in hospital may spend all day in the company of the same group of people and sleep in the same dormitory or ward at night. All his activities are regulated by the same figures of authority or the rules of the same system. If his status within such a system is one of dependency or of being subject to control then it becomes understandable that degradations, humiliations and other experiences damaging to self-concept can easily occur.

The status of a psychiatric patient within the social environment of the hospital makes him vulnerable for a number of reasons. Because he is primarily a *patient*, a barrier is created between himself and the world outside the hospital — he has a reduced range of roles available to him. He may have very few private possessions within the hospital; even his clothes and his toilet equipment may be of hospital issue. He is not safe from the intervention of others but is subject to control by drugs or other forms of therapy. He is never allowed to be alone for very long and even private activities such as dressing and undressing, sleeping and bathing are abnormally public. The staff have access to facts about himself which have had to be disclosed because he is unable to function independently but which nevertheless are intimate and often discrediting. If your colleagues knew as much about the intimate details of your life as you know about the lives of certain patients then your own self-esteem might be somewhat shaken.

Goffman describes both a pre-patient phase and an in-patient phase of the moral career and also notes the existence of an expatient phase. The pre-patient phase is concerned with the reasons for a person being admitted into hospital in the first place and the immediate effects that this has on him. Although he has been admitted in orded to be treated for some named psychiatric illness, the events leading up to this occurrence are essentially social. He is unable to cope with the demands of independent existence or other people are unable to cope with his presence or his behaviour. As Goffman puts it '*mental patients distinctively suffer not from mental disorder but from contingencies*'.

In becoming a patient he also goes through a process of redefining himself as being unbalanced or abnormal as well as receiving such labels from others. Frequently there is a member of his family, a friend or other associate who has been instrumental in getting him admitted. This person may have been partly motivated by their own inability to cope with the existing situation and partly by wanting to obtain professional help for the patient. The relationship between the patient and this 'complainant' may be damaged for two reasons. Firstly the very fact of being physically removed to a hospital disrupts or even terminates normal social relationships. Secondly the patient may have a sense of having been betrayed. The realities of hospital life and the time he will spend in hospital may have been misrepresented and he may have complied with the wishes of others in order to satisfy their immediate needs only to find himself transformed to the status of a patient with very few rights of his own.

As an in-patient the individual may first tend to disassociate himself from his surrounds but ultimately comes to accept his situation sufficiently to participate in the social life of the institution. Throughout his career as a patient his self-concept will be affected by several factors. These are the way in which he describes and presents himself and whether this version is accepted as being valid by others; the way in which he is described by others and the extent to which this is discrediting, and the physical and social environment which has been deemed a suitable background to someone of his capabilities.

The way in which an individual describes his present self, in relation to his past and his future, may normally be optimistic and place him in a favourable light. Giving an account of oneself in the middle of a busy life usually allows one to indicate some measure of success or at least the existence of a goal.

The individual who cannot account for himself except in terms of personal failure may produce either a tale of being a victim of the actions of others or an exaggerated claim to a social status, past successes or future certainties which are not entirely true. The reasons given by patients for being in hospital can often provide examples of such distortions of fact. The version a patient gives of himself may not be challenged by other inmates who cannot themselves afford to be discredited by disbelief in their own explanations. His claims are, however, likely to be disallowed by the staff whose role in the hospital includes that of enabling the patient to gain realistic views of himself and his future life. This means views which correspond with the views held by the staff and which allow him to co-operate with them.

The way in which the staff describe the patient can be illustrated by the usual content of staffroom gossip and by the typical content of case notes. This does not mean to imply that staff are hostile towards patients; they may be deeply concerned and committed to a patient's care but they still speak of the patient as an incomplete and inadequate person. His shortcomings or offences receive far more attention than his abilities or demonstrations of normal mature behaviour. This is understandable: if you take your car in for a service you don't expect the mechanic to spend all day admiring the bits that work. But if the patient is a person and not a mechanical object then these discussions between staff, which validate their own possession of knowledge and responsibility, can also be discrediting to the patient.

Case notes in particular are detailed documentations of failure, offences against society and inadequacy. Intimate details of everything that has gone wrong for an individual since infancy are collected together and added to by descriptions of his current failures, outbursts of temper or lack of co-operation. Such records are probably true and probably necessary but their existence underlines again the status that a patient holds which, amongst other things, denies him the right to withhold information about himself.

The environment of the ward in which he lives may contrast in terms of privacy, comfort and personal space with his previous experience. This deprivation is not a punishment but represents the environment with which the staff feel that the patient can cope. If he sees numbers of elderly deteriorated patients being equally able to cope with this environment then he can assess what his own capabilities are thought to be.

The patient's hospital career may involve a number of changes in status as he moves from ward to ward, between activity groups, and gains greater access to the outside world in later stages of rehabilitation.

He can move backwards as well as forwards and observes other patients doing the same. His attempts to establish a self-concept which includes being rational, successful and well are easily deflated by being reminded of his past failures or by being questioned about past events. The one thing he can learn is that however unacceptable he is in society he is always acceptable within the institution. Expectations of him are low and once he can accept a poor image of himself then it does not seem to matter. He is constantly exposed and the regard that others feel for him seems to be beyond his control. A 'moral loosening' occurs as he realizes that there is little to be lost through being observed in further indiscretions. It is true that more previleges he gains within the system the more he has to lose, but it is all a question of knowing the rules and running the risks.

Although the observations summarised here were made by Goffman in America in the early 1960s the situation of many patients has not changed so much that this picture is totally unfamiliar.

RELEVANCE TO PRACTICE

Professional attitudes

The process of normal socialization and the social situation of the patient have been the major concerns so far. However, the significance of professional education and of working as a member of staff in an essentially abnormal social environment should be mentioned, even if it cannot be discussed at length.

Professional education is a curious thing. It involves learning knowledge, skills and also a language which is subsequently used in communicating with fellow professionals. The acquisition of these features brings about certain changes in the identity of the learner: he becomes someone who can act and communicate in particular ways and who holds a qualification which has a meaning to others. In some places this identity even has a conspicuous visual part such as the wearing of a uniform.

In joining a professional group the individual comes to identify with its objectives. To an extent he accepts the doctrine upon which the group is built, learns the behaviour which is considered right or appropriate by his colleagues and uses their language and characteristic social distance in relating to others. It is quite logical that certain skills and knowledge should be defined as being a part of the equipment of one profession or another. There is so much to learn about so many things that some social distribution of knowledge is a sensible as team work is desirable.

Each profession examines and evaluates its members according to theoretical knowledge, practical ability and attitudes which it judges to be appropriate. A large number of different professions contribute towards the medical and social care of people who are disadvantaged or who require some form of service. There is inevitably an overlap of abilities and attitudes between these professional groups. Although such an overlap is to the advantage of the client, the professional groups themselves devote a great deal of energy to teaching each other, regretting that they have done so and attempting to define their own unique role. To comment on this phenomenon is not necessarily to criticize: it merely forms an example of how being a part of a professional group affects the identity of its individual members.

The maintenance of professional standards involves being monitored from within one's own professional group and also coming under the scrutiny of others who have the interests of the patients at heart. Providing a service involves coping with a number of conflicts; two examples of conflict are efficiency versus humanity and involvement versus objectivity.

To take the first: the smooth running of an occupational therapy department can be achieved by introducing systems of rules, routines and restrictions. Time and staff can be allocated to achieving set tasks and the lives of the patients ordered towards maximum efficiency. On the other hand a smoothly operating system may have been achieved at the cost of further denial of each patient's individuality and fluctuating needs. The finest organisational skills are those which are not evident and which result in an available therapist rather than a busy one. The distinction between involvement and objectivity is even more problematical. Most professions appear to frown upon emotional involvement with those whom they serve. This is probably in part for the protection of the client and in part for the protection of both therapist and colleagues. A certain social distance preserves the status of the treatment team as being different from and more complete than those who are sick. Objectivity is a necessary quality since it should not prevent a therapist from being able to empathize with individual patients but removes the confusion between empathy and sympathy, the latter being an emotional response which requires neither knowledge nor skill.

Staff distance is, of course, maintained in rather strange ways, such as not eating with patients and using separate toilets. There may be organisational reasons for such segregation but it is worth balancing these against treatment objectives of providing for patients both normal social models and opportunities for positive redefinition of self.

It would certainly be naive to believe that differences in social status between therapist and patient within an institution do not affect the nature of their relationship. The process of becoming professional is one of the ways in which this gap between each status is widened. Fortunately this does not argue that professional people should not exist or are self-defeating, only that they should offer sufficient skills and specific help to redress the balance.

Sense and semantics

This chapter has offered a lot of words and probably illustrates that there is nothing new under the sun except the words which are used to describe it. Terms such as role, socialization and status are thrown about a good deal in practice and it is worth noting that they do have more specific meanings than is sometimes realized. It is time to return to the definition of rapport given by Manford H. Kuhn and quoted at the end of Chapter 2:

> . . . it involves, at bottom, simply the sharing of a common language, so that through shared frames of reference each person in what he has to say, or in each posture he takes, calls out in himself, incipiently, the response that these gestures, postures, and symbols call out in each other.

If symbolic interaction is now the frame of reference that we share in discussing Kuhn's definition then it is clear that he is talking about role-taking or empathy. Difficulties in role-taking between therapist and patient are associated with differences in cultural background, language or vocabulary, age, sex and status or social class. We live in a relatively socially mobile society but becoming a professional worker tends to be an upward move for the individual whereas becoming a psychiatric patient is the opposite.

There are several ways in which we attempt to overcome problems of rapport. One is to use unqualified helpers whose lack of professional knowledge is counterbalanced by their ability to relate to and work alongside patients on a less threatening social basis. Another is to be so sufficiently associated with professional help that the patient can regard us as personally anoymous and useful for that reason. A third is to have sufficient insight of our own self-definition that we can recognize the problems experienced by both patients and ourselves in interaction and can allow the patient's concerns to be primary rather than the enhancement of our own identity.

Another differentiation which could be made at this point is between the performance of roles and the performance of tasks. Although what someone is has been shown to be concerned with what he can do, it is useful to make the distinction. Much of the work of the occupational therapist is concerned with teaching proficiency in a wide range of tasks. But it is possible to continue to increase a patient's ability in this respect without providing him with opportunities to practise roles other than that of learner or dependent. In college, students learn to *do* and to *know* many things but only in hospital do they learn to *be* occupational therapists. Subsequently in their departments patients may learn to perform many tasks, but only if the treatment allows them to develop positive roles within the community and their own social group can they become normal, self-respecting people.

BIBLIOGRAPHY

Becker E 1968 Socialization, command of performance, and mental illness. In: Spitzer S P, Denzin N K (eds) The mental patient, studies in the sociology of deviance. McGraw-Hill, New York
Berger P, Luckmann t 1966 the social construction of reality. Penguin, Harmondsworth
Goffman E 1961 Asylums. Essays on the social situation of mental patients and other inmates. Penguin, Harmondsworth
Goffman E 1963 Stigma. Penguin Harmondsworth

Kuhn M H 1962 The interview and the professional relationship. In: Rose A M (ed) Human behaviour and social processes. Routledge and Kegan Paul, London

Mead G H 1934 Self. In: Thompson K, Tunstall J (eds) 1971 Sociological perspectives. Penguin, Harmondsworth

Rose A M 1962 A systematic summary of symbolic interaction theory. In: Rose A M (ed) Human behaviour and social processes. Routledge and Kegan Paul, London

Sommer R, Osmond H 1962 The schizophrenic in society. Psychiatry 25: 244–255

RECOMMENDED READING

Clark D H 1974 Social therapy in psychiatry. Penguin, Harmondsworth

Cook M 1978 Perceiving others. Methuen, London

Goffman E 1959 the presentation of self in everyday life. Penguin, Harmondsworth

Manis J G, Meltzer B N 1978 Symbolic interaction, 3rd edn. Allyn and Bacon, Boston

Nelson-Jones R 1984 Personal responsibility counselling and therapy: an integrative approach. Harper and Row, London

Orford J 1976 The social psychology of mental disorder. Penguin, Harmondsworth

Rose A M (ed) 1962 Human behaviour and social processes. Routledge and Kegan Paul, London

Shaw J 1974 the self in social work. Routledge and Kegan Paul, London

Thompson K, Tunstall J (eds) 1971 Sociological prespectives. Penguin, Harmondsworth

Townsend J M 1976 Self-concept and the institutionalization of mental patients: an overview and critique. Journal of Health and Social Behaviour 17: (September) 263–271

4

Developmental approaches to treatment

The study of normal development is a natural interest for those concerned with the care of malfunctioning adults. As a parallel illustration, the study of normal anatomy and physiology is a precursor to the study of skeletal or physiological diseases or abnormalities. Some methods of treatment for brain damaged adults are based on stages of development observable in the normal child. People develop socially, emotionally and intellectually as well as physically and this can have an impact on the treatment of adults with a range of personal disabilities. The theorists selected for discussion within this chapter serve only as examples of those who have centred their concerns or therapeutic methods on development.

BASIC CONCEPTS

Development and disorder

Changes occur throughout the life of every individual. Some of these changes are attributable to physical growth and maturation, some to the acquisition of skills and some to alterations in status and social relationships. Development is most apparent in the very young when, not only is physical growth very rapid, but the range of things which a child can do, and can understand, expands continuously.

A wide range of abilities are required in order to cope, or to function effectively within the physical and social environment. These abilities can be broken down and categorised according to the stage of development to which they are appropriate. For example, the abilities required to function effectively as a 6-year-old at school are different from those required by a 65-year-old facing retirement. Reaching a specific stage in development therefore involves learning all the behaviours which are described as being part of that stage, and applying these behaviours successfully to all situations that may arise.

In the developmental view an inability to function effectively, or symptoms of psychological disturbance, arise from failures to acquire all the abilities or behaviours appropriate to the stage at which the person is attempting to operate.

These failures may be due to physical or to psycho-social factors. The mentally handicapped are disabled due to a failure in intellectual development. The reasons for this failure may be any one of the physical accidents which can affect the brain before, during or shortly after birth, but the handicap is developmental. Difficulty in establishing or maintaining normal relationships, including permanent sexual relationships, can be related to a developmental failure in childhood or adolescence. This failure may be related to psychosocial rather than physical causes. At different periods throughout life it is normal to explore and adapt a number of skills, relationships and experiences. Lack of opportunity or a repressive environment may hinder this process. For example a young person may be prevented from forming close friendships within a peer group due to conflicts or restrictions arising from his family. Under stress there is a tendency for people to regress to a lower level of functioning. This regression may be temporary or may become a feature of the way in which the individual habitually behaves.

Development as a sequential process

The study of development as a framework for treatment uses the principle that normal development is sequential. One stage or skill is established before the next can be acquired in full. There are numerous studies of normal development which demonstrate this principle. Many of these examine the different roles played by maturation and by learning, a combination of these processes appears to be essential in the development of skills and attitudes.

It would be a mistake to try to separate physical and psychological development or to differentiate between maturation and learning in introducing this topic. Any reader who feels excessively vague about normal development should revise not only the physical milestones characteristically reached in normal childhood but also look up a sequential study such as Piaget's stages of cognitive development.

Piaget, in describing the four stages of sensorimotor, pre-operational, concrete operational and formal operational cognition, demonstrates how one set of characteristics or abilities becomes integrated before a gradual transition is made to the next. Although our present subject is the treatment of psychiatrically impaired adults rather than of pre-adolescents, his distinction between concrete operational and formal operational stages is of particular interest. The concrete operational stage is characterized by logical thought and by the concept of conservation in phenomena such as quantity, mass, weight and dimension. The subject understands relationships and events within a physical and factual world. Formal operational abilities involve more abstract thinking. The subject can use hypotheses to solve problems systematically. He is concerned with values and ideology, can use similes and symbols in reasoning and in exploring abstract concepts. Some psychotic patients appear to have difficulty in applying formal operations to the solving of problems and the making of decisions. When thinking becomes disorganised as a result of illness or deterioration then interpretation becomes more rigid and learning more dependent on trial and error.

The fact that normal development is sequential has an obvious bearing on the way in which treatment can be organised to best effect. If you can assess how far an individual has travelled already on a predictable route then it should be possible to plan logical goals which are within his reach.

The schemes of development which will be summarised

here do not concentrate exclusively on the rapid changes of childhood but attempt to show the pattern of change which may occur sequentially over a normal life span. Such schemes may refer to a single dimension within a person's life such as physical strength, to give a simple example, or ego development to give a more complex one. Other schemes may be multidimensional, that is they cover a wide range of skills or functions and attempt to demonstrate the cross relationship which exists between each.

E. H. Erikson's Eight Stages of Ego Development will be used as an example of a single dimensional framework. Anne Cronin Mosey's Seven Adaptive Skills will be used as an example of the multidimensional approach.

ERIK ERIKSON'S EIGHT STAGES OF EGO DEVELOPMENT

Erik Erikson is fundamentally a neo-Freudian who was trained as an analyst in Vienna. He accepts the basic Freudian concepts of the id, the ego and the superego but his own developmental scheme concentrates on the development of the ego. His theory is termed psychosocial, whereas Freud's is psychosexual. Important relationships as desribed by Freud are centred on the family; Erikson emphasizes social processes. He relates psychological states experienced in adulthood to success or failure in resolving a series of conflicts which are met in early life. Each of his eight stages of ego development describe one of these conflicts. Successful resolution of each conflict in turn leads to an increase in the strength of the ego. A strong ego is associated with a clear sense of identity and an ability to meet further new challenges throughout life. A full description of each stage, its conflicts and consequences, is given in *Childhood and Society* (1951).

Basic trust v. basic mistrust (birth to about 1 year)

At this early age the infant learns to trust his environment. As a result of affectionate and consistent maternal care he gains confidence in the world as a predictable and continuing place in which he has 'a sense of being alright'. He also starts to have some trust in himself as control over his own body increases.

Failure to establish basic trust at this stage may arise from neglect, deprivation or other failures in maternal care. In relation to psychopathology, Erikson comments:

> The absence of basic trust can best be studied in infantile schizophrenia, while life-long underlying weakness of such trust is apparent in adult personalities in whom withdrawal into schizoid and depressive states is habitual'.

Autonomy v. shame and doubt (about 1 to 3 years)

If he is to view himself eventually as a person in his own right, separate from although still dependent on his parents, the child needs to practise being responsible for his own actions. Inevitably he will make mistakes, misjudge or misuse his own powers. He is also learning social values related to such things as nakedness and toilet training. An understanding and caring environment will support the child in establishing his autonomy and ability to make free choices. He needs the reassurance of some external control and firmness rather than to experience the chaos of anarchy. The attitudes of the parents are vital to the child if he is to gain assurance and learn to communicate. Too much punishment will lead him to experience an excess of shame and doubt.

Such excesses could have several consequences later in life; the individual may over control himself in an obsessive way, be acutely self-conscious or secretive. It is also possible that he may develop an attitude of open defiance, the feelings invoked by criticism being turned to an attack on those who pass the criticism.

Initiative v. guilt (about 4 to 5 years)

By this time the child is able, through play, to experiment in competition, co-operation and rivalry. He has increased locomotive and manipulative abilities and plenty of energy. Controls are exerted upon him not only by parents or other adults but by his own emerging superego. He may have exciting fantasies but also deeply troubling fears. If the child's early attempts at using his initiative through play are successful, or at least not squashed by punishment, he should develop a lively imagination, anticipate adult roles with confidence and have the courage to test reality with vigour. If he is over controlled, either by the intervention of others or by his imposing constrictions upon himself, then a sense of guilt may predominate.

Erikson describes an excess of guilt as leading to hysterical denial which might be expressed in physical symptoms or in an overcompensatory 'showing off'. Another outcome, where the child has over controlled himself, is the development of self-righteousness to the extent that the individual is intolerant of the initiative used by others and attempts to control them through an attitude of 'moral surveillance'.

Industry v. inferiority (from about 6 to 11 years)

Past infancy but not yet involved in adult concerns, the child is engaged in learning. He acquires formal knowledge at school and also learns to use tools. Tools include household implements, creative instruments and all the other pieces of equipment used by adults in daily life. Competence in the use of such tools is necessary both for his own benefit and in order to be a productive and contributing member of society. He learns to work co-operatively through the relationships developed in school and with young friends. Systematic learning is the major feature of a child's life during these years and, if he is successful, a sense of accomplishment and of belonging to a tool oriented society is gained. He can put play and fantasy into perspective against the identification and accomplishment of tasks.

If his attempts to learn are accompanied by a sense of failure or comparitive inferiority then the child will feel discouraged and despondent. It may be more difficult for him later in life to develop a self-concept which includes the belief that he can cope, compete and contribute within a productive world.

Identity v. role confusion (about 12 to 20 years)

This is the stage of establishing an independent identity which is so crucial to the adolescent and to the early years of being a student. Physiological development is rapid in the early part of this period but the major concern throughout is the integration of the way in which one is seen by others with the way in which one sees, and accepts, oneself. Major concerns at this stage are the acceptance and support of a peer group, identification with heroes and ideals, and the reflection and clarification of the ego through early love relationships.

The major pitfalls at this stage are, according to Erikson, doubts over sexual identity and occupational role. If you think back, most of those great traumas or arguments were about what you should do or be educated towards, and about relationships with your own and the opposite sex. Confusion as an outcome at this stage leads to problems in establishing satisfactory roles in life, in relation to work, authority, sexuality and values.

Intimacy v. isolation (early adulthood)

Establishing an identity, with some degree of confidence, prepares the young adult for taking the risk of combining that identity with another's in a lasting intimate relationship. Erikson describes the major concern as being the achievement of 'true genitality', that is, the ability to express and to experience sexuality without either damage to the ego or the use of sex as a form of combat. This is not to say that a regular sexual liaison resolves all conflict between isolation and intimacy. It is the attitude towards giving the receiving gratification which is important. Problems can lie in a retreat into isolation and prejudice which prevents the individual from being a loving person who can enjoy other people rather than fear or fight them. It is possible to remain isolated with another person in a relationship which serves mainly to protect each partner from having to face up to the next Erikson's developmental stages.

Generativity v. stagnation (middle adulthood)

Generativity means a concern for growth or for a new generation. This may involve the rearing and guidance of children but can also include other forms of productivity and creativity. To generate, in the sense of an electrical generator, is to produce energy in order to make something else work. Failure to function in this way may lead the individual to feel stagnant and impoverished and to develop a tendency towards self indulgence and hypochondria. Like the previous stage, psycho-social maturity in this sense cannot be achieved simply by fulfilling a biological function. Young parents and those without children may have equal difficulty in experiencing genuine enrichment through their own productivity.

Ego integrity v. despair (late adulthood)

Success, or a favourable ratio of the positive aspects over the negative, in the previous seven stages provides an accumulation of ego strength. This strength allows the development of a sense of perspective related to the entire life span. The individual appreciates the continuity of past, present and future of mankind, and is able to accept the pattern of his own life and his own responsibility for the way in which this pattern has emerged. The word 'integrity', like 'integrate' and 'integral', implies completeness, the bringing together of parts into a sound whole. The individual can regard the present and the future, including death, with dignity. When such personal integrity cannot be achieved, the alternative is despair. This is experienced as an accumulation of regrets and resentments. There is a feeling that, instead of bringing comfort and consolation, time has run out. With no sense of being a part of a continuing and meaningful world, impending death is frightening.

The stated purpose of summarising Erikson's eight stages of ego development was to demonstrate a single dimensional developmental scheme. But what relevance has this scheme, which concentrates largely on the conflicts of childhood, to the treatment of long term psychiatric disorders?

Erikson describes development as a process which continues throughout life. Each stage is essentially psychosocial, meaning that the inner needs of the individual are subject to the demands of the outside world. He describes each stage as having a central conflict which can have either a positive or a negative outcome. These extremes of outcome are useful in illustrating each conflict, but it should be remembered that for many people the outcome arises from the middle ground in between these extremes. Erikson emphasizes the crisis of personal identity during adolescence but a search for identity can be recognized in each of the eight conflicts. The continual development and revision of identity is the basis of self-concept which was the major theme of the last chapter. The point is that occupational therapy can, at its best, be a medium through which a personal identity can be regained and revised, and that this is a process which is relevant to any age group of patients.

It is too easy to oversimplify a developmental view of human instability but think for a moment of a stable, secure personality as being a tower built of blocks. Each developmental stage is reached and planted firmly on the smooth surface of the one that has gone before. The result is strong and balanced and will not fall down or crumble under additional weight. Very few people really fit that description. Now consider a tower that never really gets off the ground, something has gone so drastically wrong with the first few blocks that the others never got added. This is a picture of severe developmental retardation and of a person who is quite unable to function in some way. But how many people really fit that description? The third tower is one in which the blocks have somehow been piled up but their shapes are irregular and their surfaces uneven. The tower is there but the blocks are balanced precariously, the addition of each new block puts strain on the whole eccentric structure. Rather a lot of people resemble the third tower; some of them are patients and some of them are staff. We all have different degrees of instability.

Applying a development frame of reference to treatment is a matter of deciding what to do about the third tower. One alternative is to take it all to pieces and start again or at least to go back to the lowest stable block. This is one of the principles underlying Anne Cronin Mosey's approach to treatment which she calls 'Recaptitualation of ontogenesis'. Another approach is to concentrate on getting the most recent block safely in place, appreciating the eccentricity of earlier building but trying to shore the structure up enough for success to be experienced. This may sound comparatively clumsy but consider the large number of hospitalized patients in late adulthood or old age. They are still in a state of developmental crisis and the distinction between personal integrity and despair can be the major concern of those who care for them. Each patient needs every possible assistance in establishing identity and ego strength in order to strive towards a goal of personal integrity.

ANNE CRONIN MOSEY'S SEVEN ADAPTIVE SKILLS

This is a multidimensional model, that attempts to provide a developmental formula which covers all aspects of an individual's life. Developments in intellect, physical ability, social relationships and personal identity progress concurrently with each other. Mosey describes a person as having seven different aspects, each of which has its own sequence of developmental stages. The seven aspects of man relate to the seven adaptive skills. These are perceptual-motor skill, cognitive skill, drive-object skill, dyadic interaction skill, group interaction skill, self identity skill and sexual identity skill.

The first thing to qualify is the term 'adaptive'. It is not very helpful to acquire a range of skills unless their performance is both relevant and beneficial. In order to meet his own needs and those of other people an individual has to be effective within his own environment and to select and reach appropriate goals. A skill can be described as 'adaptive' if the user not only can learn it but can modify in the light of his own experiences and circumstances so that it actually works.

The developmental sequence within each of the adaptive skills is represented by a hierarchy of subskills. In most instances these are acquired in sequential order, each building on the one which has gone before. Progress in the acquisition of subskills in one skill area should have some correlation with the level of subskills attained in the others. One may use the study of different subjects at school as a rough analogy; a child may reach 'Book III' in English at about the same time as he reaches 'Book III' in Arithmetic. A patient who has difficulty in one of the adaptive skills may also have difficulty in learning skills at a corresponding level in others. For example an inability to perceive his own limitations and assets (self identity skill) may relate to an inability to interact in an authority relationship (dyadic interaction skill) or to participate in a project group (group interaction skill.)

Although Mosey's seven adaptive skills are developmentally based, and therefore considered within this chapter, this does not mean that they have nothing to do with interactionist or behavioural views. In fact both are important to understanding this frame of reference, particularly in relation to motivation. The ability to perform taks and to fulfil roles is learnt, not gained through growth. Part of the motivation for learning comes from intrinsic sources such as man's drive towards fulfulling his own needs and towards self actualization. There are also external sources of motivation, reinforcements which are forthcoming from the environment. This is an example of a frame of reference used in treatment which draws from more than one theoretical base. Such interdependence of different theoretical concepts is one of the themes of the next chapter.

The adaptive skills

The intention here is to summarise, and perhaps clarify, what is meant by each adaptive skill. There is insufficient space to discuss the content of every subskill under each heading. If it is helpful to return to the analogy of the building blocks, then visualise seven towers being built so close to each other that they form part of the same structure. Being interdependent for support, each tower is added to at approximately the same rate if the resulting structure is to be solid and sound.

Perceptual-motor skill

This hierarchy of subskills is concerned with the ability to perceive a variety of sensory stimuli and to respond to them appropriately. It involves the ability to use knowledge about the properties of external objects and to plan gross and fine motor movements. An example of using perceptual-motor skills can be as simple as picking up a pencil. Your eye can tell you exactly where it is in relation to other objects, you know that it is solid, inflexible and light in weight, your arm and your fingers obey precise commands to reach out, grasp and retrieve it. This sounds very easy but a small child needs to learn to discriminate stimuli and to control action to such a fine degree. I still cannot listen to a series of notes played on the piano and then persuade my vocal cords to reproduce them exactly.

Cognitive skill

Literally the ability to think, this skill is concerned with being able to process and to use information. Objects or stimuli are perceived and understanding of them is stored away for later use. If such information has later to be represented in some way, it may be as a movement, a pictorial image or as an abstract idea. For example, three different fishermen are asked about a fish that each of them has caught. One may indicate the size of the fish by spacing his hands apart or mime the effort of landing it, this is a representation through motor movement. The second may represent pictorially by describing the visual image of the fish as he still 'sees' it in his mind, its comparative size and its appearance. The third may represent the fish in terms of the feelings that it invoked in him. Such a representation may be hard to communicate because it is difficult, for most people, to put feelings into words or pictures without losing some of the meaning.

Having perceived and represented objects or events in these ways, the information still needs to be organised in order to be useful. The subskills in this area are concerned with degrees of ability to recognise cause and effect, to select information, to solve problems in different ways and to communicate with other people using abstract ideas.

Drive-object skill

A drive is the energy that the individual puts into satisfying his needs. These needs are outlined within the discussion of Maslow's work in the second chapter. Certain 'objects' will either help an individual to satisfy his needs or will hinder him in his attempts to do so. Some objects may be non-human, for example buildings, tools, books, animals, materials or the weather. Helpful objects may be things like a sharp chisel, a clear set of instructions or a willing horse.

Other objects can be unhelpful, like a jar that will not open, an icy road or a refrigerator which irritates by humming and juddering all day. Human objects are of course people, and in different ways they can be helpful or unhelpful too. In addition to human and non-human objects, abstract ideas and values can help or hinder an individual's drive to fulfil his needs. Adherence to a particular set of beliefs or ideals may enable some one to feel esteemed or accepted. Conversely they may prevent him from pursuing certain goals.

The drive-object skill is the ability to co-ordinate personal drives with existing objects. In order to be successful in satisfying needs, some drives may have to be controlled and some objects particularly selected or avoided. The degree to which an individual can form a useful relationship between personal drives and existing objects is the basic of each subskill.

Dyadic interaction skill

Whenever two are met together, that is a dyadic interaction. The relationship that can develop between those two people depends upon the participating skills of each. The basic requirement is for each to recognise the other as being unique and separate and to be willing to associate with him. There are many different relationships possible between two people, such as friendship, authority, intimacy, caring and being cared for. The level of relationship that an individual is able to enter into depends on the level of subskills which he has attained. The ability to commit oneself to a mutually satisfying intimate relationship requires a higher level of subskills than the type of sharing and trust which character- ises what Mosey terms a 'chum relationship'.

Group interaction skill

Like relationships between two people, groups differ in quality according to the skills and the maturity of the partic- ipants. The least demanding group is one in which members are all physically present and acting in parallel with each other but not necessarily in active co-operation. A group usually has a common purpose and its members share certain interests and abilities. One person may belong to several different groups and skills are required to make the membership of each productive and satisfying. Skills include those of communicating ideas, reaching decisions and goals in co-operation with other people, accepting and adapting to the norms of behaviour established by the group and helping to resolve problems. In order to participate effectively an individual must learn to adopt different roles within the group and to see things from the point of view of others. Mosey defines the attainment of subskills by the maturity of the group in which an individual is able to function effectively.

Self identity skill

Self identity or self-concept is becoming a rather recurrent theme so it seems superfluous to offer yet another definition. Mosey's concept of self identity relates very closely to the interactionist views discussed in Chapter 3. In determining subskills, she describes perceptions of self developing through recognition of being separate, having individual attributes and responsibilities, being part of a social reality and accepting change and aging.

Sexual identity skills

The prior reading of Erikson's eight stages in ego development should have indicated the importance of the development of sexuality in establishing both satisfactory roles in life and also a strong sense of personal identity and values. Mosey defines the mature sexual identity skill as 'the ability to perceive one's sexual nature as good and to participate in a heterosexual relationship which is oriented to the mutual satisfaction of sexual needs'. The subskills are concerned with the acceptance of one's own sexuality and of physiological development and needs. Sexuality can be rejected, can be selfishly orientated or can be an expression of deep concern for another's pleasure as well as one's own. At the other end of the scale of physiological development is a decline in sexual desires and activity. The ultimate skill is to be able to accept these changes without a deterioration in the concept of either oneself or one's sexual partner.

Recapitulation of ontogenesis

Having described the seven adaptive skills Mosey offers a model of treatment which is based on these developmental concepts. This model is 'Recapitulation of ontogenesis'. To recapitulate is to go over again and ontogenesis in this context means one's own developmental process.

It is first of all accepted that, whatever condition the patient is said to be suffering from, his actual problems arise from his position on a developmental road between a state of function and a state of dysfunction. Milestones on this road are marked by the attainment of subskills in each of the adaptive skill areas. In order to plan the treatment of a patient two assessments have to be made. The first is of the patient's current developmental status in each adaptive skill. This means identifying which subskills have already been learnt and are being applied successfully. The second is of the demands of whatever environment the patient is expected to settle in. This might be a sheltered environment or one in which all the pressures which existed prior to hospitalisation are again present. This involves identifying the level of subskills in each adaptive skill area which will be needed by the patient if he is going to be able to cope.

Assessment of the patient in each of the seven adaptive skills can be attempted in different ways. For example standardised tests may be available to determine his ability in perceptual motor skills. Most of the information however arises from the therapist's observation of the patient while he is engaged in relevant tasks or interactions with other people. The patient can give direct information about the levels which he has reached in discussing his own needs and abilities. Indirect information can also be gained from discussion by noticing the words that he uses to describe himself and other people and the way in which he represents ideas.

The subskills are arranged in a hierarchical order so that, once his present level of functioning has been established, the next subskill in the sequence becomes the immediate treatment goal. Treatment starts by tackling the next subskill in the area in which he is most deficient and then may move to include deficient areas from other adaptive skills. The idea is first to bring the seven towers of building blocks level with each other before increasing the overall height of the structure.

There are two main ways in which the patient is helped to attain his next sequential subskill. The first is through providing a 'growth-facilitating environment'. This means making sure that the situation in which the patient is placed provides opportunities for learning the behaviours appropriate to the subskill which he is trying to attain. For example, if the subskill is the ability to participate in a co-operative group then he should be placed with compatible people who are developmentally ready to work together in this way, and who will reinforce each other for participating effectively. The second way of helping the patient is through the direct application of methods based on learning theory. The patient's behaviour is shaped towards the attainment of the subskill by the positive reinforcement of behaviours which are compatible with the subskill.

This approach to treatment is presented in a logical and comprehensive way. Occupational therapists are divided, in some parts of the world, as to whether it provides a solution to the problems inherent in the rehabilitation of psychiatric patients, or whether it provides an opportunity to worry about words instead of worrying about people. It is perhaps advisable to study the concepts in detail within the work of Anne Cronin Mosey and to observe their application within the occupational therapy department of a psychiatric unit before venturing an opinion.

BIBLIOGRAPHY

Ausubel D P, Kirk D 1977 Ego psychology and mental disorder. Grune and Stratton, New York

Erikson E H 1965 Childhood and society, revised edn. Triad/Paladin, St Albans

Hall C S, Lindzey G 1970 Theories of personality, 2nd edn. John Wiley, New York

Mosey A C 1970 Three frames of reference for mental health. Charles B. Slack, Thorofare, New Jersey

Mosey A C 1973 Activities therapy. Raven Press, New York

Shaw J 1974 The self in social work. Routledge and Kegan Paul, London

RECOMMENDED READING

Beard R M 1969 An outline of Piaget's developmental psychology.
    Routledge and Kegan Paul, London
Boyle D G 1969 A student's guide to Piaget. Pergamon Press, Oxford
Cohen J, Clarke J 1979 Medicine mind and man. Freeman, Reading
Schuster C S, Ashburn S S 1980 The process of human development. Little
    & Brown, Boston
Weinemann J 1981 An outline of psychology as applied to medicine. John
    Wright, Bristol

5

A brief perspective

Is all this theoretical background really necessary? This brief addition to the previous four chapters will indicate some of the reasons why the answer has to be 'yes'. It would also be useful to clarify what has been achieved so far, how it all fits together and how it gives indications for treatment.

SEMANTICS AGAIN

The phrase 'approach to treatment' is particularly useful since it neatly avoids differentiation between theories, models and frames of reference. These three terms, each of which occurs in the preceding chapters, do overlap to an extent. Some attempt, however, should be made to sort them out.

Theory

A theory offers an explanation of the relationship between events. Consider as an example the work of a learning theorist such as Thorndike (1911). He explained that learning occurs only when the response has some effect on the environment. If this effect is unpleasant then the behaviour is weakened but if it is pleasant then learning occurs and the behaviour is more likely to be repeated. It so happened that his experiments concerned the behaviour of cats, but if his theory is generally applicable then the same relationship between events should be observable in the behaviour of other animals, as of course has been demonstrated.

If a theory explains how things happen, or in what circumstances they happen, then it should be possible to test it experimentally in different ways and consistently arrive at a similar outcome. Once sufficient evidence has been accumulated to support the theory then it can be used to make predictions. For example, if positive reinforcement makes a behaviour more likely to be repeated, then rewarding a patient for promptness should make him more likely to be punctual. Alfred Schutz (1954) suggested that the word 'theory' 'means in all empirical sciences the explicit formulation of determinate relations between a set of variables in terms of which a fairly extensive class of empirically ascertainable regularities can be explained.'

Schutz was writing in the context of the social sciences in which the collection of empirical data can cause problems, since 'empirical' means based on experiment or directly observable. Although it is possible to observe or measure people's actions and their physical state, it is more difficult to regard mood, attitude and ideas as empirical evidence in the same way. The study of personality and of mental illness is affected by these problems since it depends to a large extent on the study of individuals and on interpretation. It is therefore not surprising that a wide range of theories have resulted, many of which overlap with each other rather than being in competition. The popularity of behaviourism may be largely due to the respectability which it gives to psychology as an empirical science. It explains empirically ascertainable regularities in a consistent way, arguments tend to be centred on the ethics of its application rather than on whether it is true or not.

Theories of personality and theories related to the possible causes of mental illness run into difficulties additional to those of empirical evidence. There are often too many known and unknown variables. For example, attempts to relate the onset of schizophrenia to particular aspects of early family life have established some links but findings tend to be inconsistent and do not always allow for a genetic factor or for other possibly significant elements.

Model

A model is usually based on one or more theories and is similar in that it offers links between different concepts or events. These links, however, are not proposed in order to be empirically tested but are intended to guide understanding and action. Refer back to Chapter 1 and you will find a section on 'Learning theory' followed by a section on 'The structure of behavioural treatment'. The first provides an explanation of how it works and the second gives a model from which treatment can be devised.

Many models, from wiring diagrams to training in social skills, can be represented pictorially. Figure 5.1 is a much simplified model of treatment.

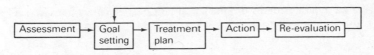

Figure 5.1 Simplified model of treatment

The advantage of such a model is that each person involved in its implementation can identify and discuss the current task whilst having a clear idea of what they should be doing next.

A model can also provide a framework for analyzing ideas or behaviour. A model in this sense can be a series of concepts or actions arranged in a pattern which is thought to be typical. One example is that of describing human inter-action in terms of games. Anatol Rapoport (1960) describes social strategies by suggesting that an individual makes certain moves, as one would in chess, selecting from alterna-tives in order to gain a satisfactory 'pay off' for himself. Eric Berne (1964) uses a similar analogy in describing the dis-honesties and strategies which occur within social relationships. Transactional analysis arises, as a model from these ideas. The basic concept is that each individual can choose to operate from one of three basic positions, 'parent', 'adult' or 'child'. Each of these three can be further subdivided and elaborated upon. In any transaction with another person communication may be complementary, for example adult to adult or parent to child and child to parent, or it may be crossed in that one person is using perhaps an adult to adult channel but the response is child to parent or some other variation. There is no intention to explain the complexities and application of transactional analysis here but Figure 5.2 shows how typical patterns of interaction can be represented in an interactionist model which can be used to explore and understand what is happening.

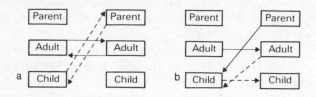

Figure 5.2 Typical patterns of interaction (a) Complementary transactions (b) Crossed transactions

Frame of reference

There is little to distinguish a frame of reference from a 'model' within psychiatric treatment. The terms have grown to popularity in different parts of the world but both essentially provide a structure upon which action can be based as opposed to theories which describe and explain how things work. The phrase 'frame of reference' appears to be used in two ways within current literature. The first usage is similar to the meaning of 'model' in that it implies a system of rules which direct a method of going about something or of interpreting events. The national grid is a frame of reference if you happen to want to pinpoint your exact geographical location on a map. 'Social skills training' is a frame of reference if you want to plan and explain group activities in a certain way.

The other use of 'frame of reference' is to embrace the theory along with the patterns of its practical application. In this way one might refer to a behavioural frame of reference as including both learning theory and the use of techniques for modifying behaviour and expect someone who shares the same background knowledge to understand what one is doing. To this extent a frame of reference becomes a common language since those who share knowledge of certain concepts can implement and communicate them without entering into lengthy explanations or justifications.

Unfortunately the suggested explanation of terms given here does not solve the problems likely to be met in more comprehensive reading. What one person calls a theory another will refer to as a model, a frame of reference or, even worse, a theoretical framework. In Chapter 3 'interactionist theory' was discussed but it it not, strictly speaking, a theory at all. It provides a structure and a language for appreciating the dynamics of communication but does not set up a hypothesis to be proved or disproved by empirical testing.

Do not despair, the important thing to decide about each piece of knowledge is whether it is useful or not. There are many contradictory assertions about the nature of social reality: theoretical research helps in differentiating between fact and fiction. Even if occupational therapy is not in itself an empirical science there is no justification for basing therapeutic measures on fiction.

THE MEDICAL MODEL

If there is something wrong with your body then you may take it to a medical practitioner and ask to have the problem diagnosed and treated. The structure of concepts which make up a medical model include those of deciding which of the known conditions an individual is suffering from on the basis of his history and symptoms, and treating him accordingly. This obviously works efficiently in physical medicine since a correct diagnosis should lead to the medical team being able to treat the condition centrally or to apply drugs or other methods to relieve the symptoms without obscuring their understanding of what is causing them. This is the traditional and tested model of a discipline whose historical development has been parallel to the development of knowledge about the pathology and treatment of physical disorders.

The application of a medical model to psychiatric conditions is a subject of considerable debate. The ideas of R. D.

Laing and the 'antipsychiatry' school were mentioned within Chapter 2. Thomas S. Szasz (1972) argues that there can be no such thing as mental illness since disease and illness by definition can only affect the body. The progress of psychiatry is hindered by outmoded concepts and terminology which persist in categorising sick people and equipping practitioners with an understanding of physical sciences rather than of communication. Szasz concludes that 'There is no medical, moral or legal justification for involuntary psychiatric interventions, such as "diagnosis", "hospitalization", or "treatment". They are crimes against humanity'.

It is necessary to balance views such as this against circumstances which favour the employment of a medical model. Organic conditions which manifest themselves in disturbed behaviour such as senile or presenile dementias and confusion arising from chemical toxins or deficiencies benefit from a diagnostic approach. Failure to make a correct differential diagnosis may prevent or delay effective treatment. Unfortunately, knowledge of the causes of mental distress is far from complete. Antidepressant drugs or, more controversially, electro convulsive treatment may help to relieve some of the symptoms of depressive illness just as the use of major tranquillizers reduces the outwardly manifested agitations of psychoses. This is, however, symptomatic treatment; the measures taken do not reflect total understanding of the underlying cause of disturbance nor do they effect a cure.

Another pertinent factor is the possibly negative effect of labelling. This was discussed briefly in Chapter 3. An individual who is perceived as being sick, particularly if this perception includes a diagnostic categorization, will have difficulty in perceiving himself as normal. Additionally, members of the medical team will tend to interpret all his behaviour in the light of the label which he has been given.

This debate can be left for now to the medical practitioners to whom it must be a central concern. Our problem is whether the medical model is useful to occupational therapy. There are certainly reasons why we should be familiar with this model: if it is being applied by others to patients who are receiving occupational therapy then communication throughout the treatment team is likely to be based on its associated language and terminology. It is also important to appreciate the possible response or side effects experienced by patients who are receiving a variety of treatments.

On the other hand occupational therapy is based on the problems experienced by an individual and not on his diagnostic label. Activities which may benefit a patient are not prescribed on the basis of his specified 'illness'. For example, if a man is learning to cook a meal for himself in the occupational therapy department the likely reason is to give him confidence in his ability to prepare food. One does not cook because one is schizophrenic nor paint because one has a depressive illness.

SUMMARY

Each of the preceding chapters considered one perspective from which patients and their treatment can be viewed.

The behavioural view is based on learning theory and the concept that all patterns of behaviour are learnt or shaped by patterns of reinforcement. This is a useful source of reference for occupational therapy since it is based on observable behaviour and activity. Occupational therapists primarily work through providing and teaching different forms of activity. This does not preclude a concern for a patient's self-concept; it is what a patient is able to do which forms a major influence on the way he views himself and the way others view him.

Humanistic views or phenomenology concentrate on an individual's perception of the world and of his part in it. He is essentially responsible for his own actions and seeks both to satisfy his own needs and to fulfil his own potential as a complete person. His success in doing this and the experience which he gains along the way will determine the value which he places on himself and the confidence with which he can relate to others. The numerous therapeutic methods which have arisen from this school of thought include not only Rogerian client-centred therapy but also Gestalt therapy, reality therapy and transactional analysis. These latter approaches have not been discussed since their application is not specific to the rehabilitation of long term patients. However, the basic concepts of this school of thought have been included because they stress the right of each individual to determine his own existence and destiny. We are reminded that any patient is primarily a unique individual rather than an interesting collection of behaviours and 'symptoms'.

Symbolic interaction has been included as an excursion into a socio-cultural view. It examines the social relationship between an individual and the other people who influence him. These others may be either specific individuals or a culture or group to which the belongs. The nature of the interaction between himself and this socio-cultural background find expression in his social status and self concept. This obviously has links with a humanistic view of man. It was selected as a topic here, in preference to describing the phenomenological treatment models mentioned above, because it usefully defines terms already used within occupational therapy and because it gives indications for the use of the social environment in a therapeutic way and for the development of community care.

Developmental approaches to treatment provide an opportunity to relate problems or abilities to a normal sequence of stages. This not only provides another explanation of how, and perhaps when, things go wrong but also suggests a sequentially structured design for programmes of treatment. This is perhaps the closest we have come to psychoanalytic theory which is the one major influence on therapy to be omitted in this book. The reason for this omission is that related techniques such as group psychotherapy, psychodrama and the projective use of the arts are not being included either, since their principal use is not with the group of patients under consideration.

These perspectives on the practice of therapy are not mutually exclusive, in fact it is difficult to centre practice on one theoretical base without at least acknowledging the influence of others. For example, training in social skills is essentially behavioural since it is concerned with the acquisition of particular behaviours through modelling, rehearsal and reinforcement. However it is motivated and directed by a humanistic view, equipping an individual to explore and fulfil himself within a social world. A recapitulation of ontogenesis, described by Mosey, draws from interactionist and learning theory although it is based on a developmental framework.

The model of treatment adopted will depend to a large

extent on the ethos of the hospital or unit concerned since the occupational therapist should be an integrated member of a multidisciplinary team providing treatment. An eclectic approach, that is one which draws from more than one theory, is frequently used. Eclecticism does, however, require action to be based on knowledge; the term does not cover a general mix up of ideas and activities which cannot be justified in any way. Given a problem or a set of problems, an occupational therapist should be able to devise a method of intervention which can be related back to tested theories or models, explained clearly to others and is amenable to some form of evaluation.

BIBLIOGRAPHY

Berne E 1964 Games people play. Penguin, Harmondsworth
Bolles R C 1975 Learning theory. Holt, Rinehart and Winston, New York
Mosey A C 1970 Three frames of reference for mental health. Charles B. Slack, New Jersey
Rapoport A 1960 Fights, games and debates. Ann Arbor, University of Michigan
Schutz A 1954 Concept and theory formation in the social sciences. In: Thompson K, Tunstall J 1971 (eds) Sociological perspectives. Penguin, Harmondsworth
Szasz T S 1972 The myth of mental illness. Paladin, St Albans
Thorndike E L 1911 Animal intelligence. Macmillan, New York

RECOMMENDED READING

Clare A 1976 Psychiatry in dissent, 2nd edn. Tavistock, London
Innes W 1981 Psychiatry: a confused profession. Pupuke Press, Auckland
Kleinmuntz B 1980 Essentials of abnormal psychology. Harper and Row, San Fransisco
Reed K, Sanderson R 1980 Concepts of occupational therapy. William and Wilkins, Baltimore
Woolams S, Brown M 1979 T A — the total handbook of transactional analysis. Prentice-Hall, Englewood Cliffs, New Jersey

PART TWO

The structure of therapy

6

The patients

LONG-TERM CARE

It is almost impossible to use diagnostic terms to categorize all those who may need psychiatric care during lengthy periods of their lives. Each patient has his own complex reasons for not being able to cope independently within society. These reasons may stem from organic impairment, from the manifestations of psychosis, from social pressures or from long standing personal inadequacy. In order to keep this chapter brief some knowledge of general psychiatry must be assumed on the part of the reader. The purpose here is to focus on particular problems, or on knowledge especially pertinent to the occupational therapist, rather than to provide any detailed description of the conditions or problems mentioned.

Wing & Morris (1981) provide the following information about the problem which faces us now and in the future:

> At the end of 1976, there were 83 939 in-patients in English psychiatric hospitals (1.81 per 1000 general population). Of these 43 per cent were men and 57 per cent women. Nearly half of the total (49 per cent) were aged 65 years or more. Only 32 per cent had been in hospital for less than a year, while 46 per cent had been resident for more than five years; the remaining 22 per cent having relatively recently become 'long

stay'. Those who have stayed for a very long time in hospital are therefore increasingly elderly and frail.

Wing & Morris go on to mention that in the same year some 15 000 people were currently attending day hospital or day centres and estimate, on the basis of the Camberwell register, a figure of:

> 420 people per 100 000 (210 000 nationally) who, at the end of 1976 had been in touch with psychiatric service for more than a year, including a spell in some kind of residential or day accommodation.

Figures given for 1976 may feel out of date at the time of reading but they do give a very real appreciation of the psychiatric population which confronts us now and which is tending to produce more and more elderly people in need of special care.

Three particularly interesting facts arise from the available statistics. Firstly that a large proportion of the existing population of psychiatric patients are elderly and that the remainder inevitably, are aging. Secondly, that over 40% of the long stay patients have been given a diagnosis of schizophrenia. Thirdly that, despite the intensive efforts in the 1960s and 1970s to rehabilitate psychiatric patients into the community, in an effort eventually to make redundant the large old psychiatric hospitals, a 'new chronic population' still appears to be arising from current admissions. The majority of these are either elderly ladies or schizophrenics. These different factors contribute to a situation where services will need to cater for both very handicapped people who have problems related to having been within institutions for many years and for newly admitted patients who need to be guarded as far as possible from the negative influences of institutionalism.

Institutionalism

This term is used to describe the effects on the individual of long-term care as opposed to the effects of the primary condition or problem which caused him to receive treatment in the first place. For those using a variety of texts, the terms 'institutionalism', 'institutionalization' and 'institutional neurosis' are roughly synonymous.

The severely institutionalized patient is recognizable by a range of well known features. He has few personal possessions and shows little concern for his appearance, he is compliant with the hospital's routine and allows all aspects of his life to be controlled by others, and he has a poor sense of time beyond mealtimes. He expects and receives little privacy, for example picking his nose or scatching his balls without regard for who may be watching. He makes no plans, showing little regard for his own future and even less for that of others. He may stoop, shuffle or move about slowly and with no apparent purpose and may spend long periods leaning against radiators or smoking for physical comfort. Although displaying little emotion he appears muscularly tense rather than relaxed. This catalogue of unhappy examples belongs to the acute syndrome and is not always typical of those who are less seriously affected.

We are all vulnerable to the effects of being part of an institution. Even college students, who drop into the habit of complying without question with regulations, timetables and philosophies which are imposed on them in the name of education, can become both regimented and apathetic. Staff working within hospitals or day centres can become dependent on hierarchies and routines rather than maintaining or developing the ability to think for themselves.

These concepts should be familiar from the brief revue of Erving Goffman's work in Chapter 3. Essentially the roles available to a patient are eroded by the adoption by staff of responsibility for his behaviour and welfare and by his status as a psychiatric patient. Institutionalism is essentially a sociological concept; it arises from a social environment or from the breakdown of normal social behaviour and responsibilities. Schizophrenic patients may be particularly vulnerable to the effects of social poverty since there are features of schizophrenia, as an experience, which reduce the quality or the quantity of social contact even when a normal range of roles and environments is available to the patient.

THE ELDERLY

Normal expectations

Each of us will either die at a comparatively young age or will grow old. If the former is regarded as a misfortune then it is a pity to be equally gloomy about aging as the alternative. There are many myths surrounding old age which are reinforced by the imbalanced concepts which one can acquire by working in close contact with the degenerative aspects of aging. Being old does not always involve being either handicapped or dependent. Remember, for example, the Gruenberg study of 1961 which showed that, at that date, over 70% of those above the age of 85 years were free from the severe effects of mental deterioration. Neither should we be too glib in referring to inevitably failing intellectual power. It is difficult to be sure that standard methods of testing intelligence are valid when used with elderly people. Tests which measure speed of response may show a decline but this does not necessarily mean that the 'power' or quality of reasoning is less adequate. Old people can only be said to be *different* from younger ones. For example they bring to bear different values on problems, different concepts of self and of society, more experience and less haste. At this end of life it is impossible to predict a person's performance on the basis of his chronological age. Some 95-year-olds are able to live independently and others, for a variety of reasons, need physical and social support at the age of 70.

Attitudes held by younger people towards the elderly inevitably affect the roles that the latter are able to fulfil, and their own concepts of themselves and of society. If, between the ages of 20 and 40, you were to lose your spouse, your siblings, significant friends and even your children, this would be recognised as being a dramatic sequence of traumas. Other people would probably react by being shocked, sympathetic and supportive. Such a sequence of events is the common experience of many old people who are expected to have the internal resources to cope with the personal and social consequences of multiple bereavement. If the elderly sometimes appear somewhat inflexible in their values, this does not always have to be interpreted in terms of physiological deterioration. It can be graceless in the young to be intolerant of ideas or practices which have proved their effectiveness in the context of an old person's history and experience.

Retirement, or increased freedom from family responsibilities, can produce problems in adjusting to changes in status and circumstances, but can also bring opportunities. Such opportunities include developing interests, spending more time with particular friends and having an active part to play as a grandparent. Old people tend to choose to spend more time reflecting on past events and on current problems. Adapting to physical changes and reviewing and accepting the course of one's own life are important parts of attaining the integrity described by Erikson as the positive outcome of the last developmental dilemma.

Active involvement within events and relationships correlates with a high morale and an ability to adapt to aging (Madox, 1963). In many cultures old people have specific roles and responsibilities within a family or social hierarchy and are particularly respected. Culture and tradition can be a focus of interest and involvement for the elderly, providing not only activity but also a perspective which gives meaning to their own lives.

Problems related to aging

The difficulties affecting an old person may be as a result of physical change or disease, of mental illness or emotional disturbance, of social conditions or stress or of increased vulnerability to long standing problems. Although, to an extent, these causes can be considered separately, in reality they are often closely interlinked. For example, a physical handicap which reduces mobility will affect social opportunity. Social isolation or being made to feel a nuisance to others can contribute towards depression or anxiety. Those who are depressed are more likely to neglect their physical health and fail to make efforts to fulfil their social needs. This rather simplistic sketch of how vicious circles can be created should also indicate that the treatment of one problem, without recognition of the others, can be ineffective.

Physical changes affect every system of the body. Cardiovascular changes may render the heart less efficient or less able to react well to sudden stress; alternatively arteriosclerosis may develop and eventually reduce the supply of oxygenated blood to the cerebral cortex. Pulmonary changes may result in an older person becoming breathless more quickly in response to exercise and in increased vulnerability to infections of the lower respiratory tract. Musculoskeletal changes affect posture and gait. There is little point here in continuing the catalogue of metabolic, endocrine, gastrointestinal or genitourinary changes, all of which can cause trouble or inconvenience. This is not a textbook on physical medicine, but nor are mentally disturbed old people disembodied head cases.

Sensory impairments are of particular importance since effective vision and hearing are vital to being able to receive, process and respond to stimuli. Defective hearing is particularly isolating and can lead not only to depressive reactions but also to the development of suspicion, hostility and apparently psychotic behaviour.

Psychiatric conditions which appear in old age may be due to changes in the central nervous system or may have more social origins. Within the central nervous system a general reduction in electrical activity may cause slower or altered sensory reception and delayed response. This is why a younger mind often has to wait for an older one to grasp fully what is happening now. Actual damage to the tissue of the brain, which may be gradual in, for example, arteriosclerosis or abrupt as in a cerebrovascular accident, has more serious consequences. Gradual but significant deterioration after the age of 65, known as senile dementia, can be compared with the speeded up effects of normal aging. It is true that both involve the loss of functional ability, but senile dementia appears to have qualitative as well as quantitative effects on performance. Disintegration of the personality accompanies loss of physical, intellectual and emotional controls. Of course it is difficult to make comparisons with normal aging processes since so few normal people exceed the age of 100. Perhaps by the age of a 130 we would all be displaying symptoms of confusion, helplessness, incontinence, emotional lability and catastrophic reaction.

The social origins of distress in the elderly are not difficult to identify. Many of these are associated with loss and bereavement. Spouses and contemporaries die, freedom of movement is lost through physical handicap, status is lost through retirement or disengagement from the family. Loneliness can be increased by younger members of the family moving away, by sensory impairment, rehousing and lack of facilities or transport. Poverty can lead to poor nutrition, inadequate heating and lack of social recreation. It is not surprising that so many old people are depressed. Meyer in 1977 even suggested that depression may be a normal reaction to aging. Some old people respond to stress by becoming very agitated or anxious, some by drinking, by misusing drugs or by neglecting themselves. The complicated range of symptoms which results can make it difficult to differentiate between a social consequence and an organic problem.

To relate depression with social causes implies that depression should be regarded as essentially reactive rather than as having a physiological base. A closer study of psychiatry will reveal debates about reactive depression as opposed to endogenous depression or psychotic depression or manic depressive psychoses. This is a fascinating area of study and has direct bearing on the prescription of drugs or other physical treatments. Other theories relate depression to genetic predisposition or to 'learned helplessness'. Whatever the biological, behavioural or environmental factors the result is someone who is actutely miserable, unable to cope with life and who could be suicidal.

Growing old in hospital

Not all elderly patients are suffering from conditions which have occurred during, or as a consequence of, their advanced age. Presenile dementias by definition occur prior to normal aging. Huntington's chorea occurs as a genetically determined form of dementia with a relatively early onset. Depressive illness of long standing may persist and worsen during old age. Schizophrenic patients age like the rest of us and, if they are living in hospital, may add syndromes of gradually increasing dependence to their problems. Whatever your problem or your diagnostic label you will grow old with it. The mentally handicapped, thanks to antibiotics, grow old and the staff who treat them grow old.

There are very few psychiatric conditions which people spontaneously grow out of; in fact institutional care can often result in growing into one's classification. For those patients for whom discharge is not contemplated some very special problems arise. Can they retire from being treated through industrial therapy or other structured activities? How can increasing physical dependence be prevented from causing a decrease in privacy and respect? Does their status as psychiatric patients include provision of regular tests of vision and hearing, chiropody, hairdressing, library or leisure interests? It is in this area that the hackneyed phrase 'quality of life' becomes pertinent. None of the professional staff involved can afford the luxuries of either apathy or despair until they are quite sure that what is being provided would be appropriate to their own parents or grandparents should they be similarly disadvantaged.

Old people, whatever their condition, are increasingly territorial. They like their own place with their possessions consistently arranged. There is a favourite chair or a habitual route for walking along the boundary. Familiarity is reassuring and every habitual practice, however odd to outsiders, is probably based on some reason or need. Being transferred from a familiar environment to a hospital is traumatic at any age but can be particularly distressing and confusing to the aged. Wisely, such a measure is avoided whenever possible by those who are trying to conserve the patient's independence and clarity of thought. When it is necessary, for medical or for social reasons, staff need to be very supportive and to accept that the patient may be experiencing anxiety, loss and confusion. If the result of this is a tendency for the patient to wander, mentally or physically, then real care may involve wandering with him.

SCHIZOPHRENIA

Those who have been given the diagnostic label of schizophrenia comprise by far the largest group in current receipt of long-term psychiatric care. There is, however, considerable debate about the cause of this condition, its variations, its treatment, and even its existence. An occupational therapist who is interested in treating 'schizophrenic' patients should be equally interested in the many different views which have been expressed. The student will probably start with the psychiatric text book description of schizophrenia as a disease with a number of possible origins and will progress to wanting to know more about the problems and challenges which these patients provide. The notes given here must presume basic text book knowledge but are intended to awake further curiosity.

A summary

A number of different classifications have been used in the past to divide patients within the group termed schizophrenic. Simple, hebephrenic, catatonic, paranoid and other types have been described, each with their own typical onset, features and prognosis. A slightly simpler view attempts to identify only two major categories, the 'process' schizophrenic whose entire life history contains episodes or evidence of being different from other people, and the 'reactive' schizophrenic who appears to have a normal developmental history into adult life but who responds to stress by producing acute psychotic symptoms. The illness of the latter type, also referred to as 'schizophreniform illness', although severe and sometimes bizarre in presentation, can respond better to treatment since the personality may be relatively intact.

Psychotic impairment where paranoia is the dominating feature is often classified separately. The paranoid schizophrenic may retain organisation of perception and of personality although he interprets the social world as hostile to himself.

There are many theories related to the cause of schizophrenia. Although genetic, biochemical and social influences can each be demonstrated as having considerable significance, no one factor has yet been isolated as being uniquely responsible. It is quite possible that a combination of such influences meet in an individual who subsequently becomes unable to manage normally. If one discrete cause could be identified, this would of course simplify the further debate regarding treatment. At present psychotrophic drugs, in particular the phenothiazine derivatives, combined with social methods, tend to dominate the scene. Psychosurgery is rarely attempted in this context, and electroconvulsive treatment has failed to justify itself as a routine method of treatment for these patients.

Because of the wide varieties of ways in which a schizophrenic patient may present himself, and because of an awareness of the inherent dangers of diagnostic labelling, many psychiatrists are wary of using the term 'schizophrenia' at all. Such difficulties are compounded by political, philosophical, or perhaps simply regional differences. Sartorius et al (1974), carrying out the International Pilot Study of Schizophrenia, showed that although a core of schizophrenics presenting first rank symptoms would be similarly diagnosed in any of the nine countries studied, the more marginal cases would be differently diagnosed in different places. The most inclusive concept of schizophrenia were found in the United States and in the Soviet Union. In other European and eastern centres the same patients would be equally likely to be diagnosed as personality disorders, neurotic, manic or depressed.

Any research or discussion such as this requires at least a proposed definition of schizophrenia as a medical condition. Clare (1976) describes three 'first rank' symptoms of the condition, without which the diagnosis would be unjustified.

1. Passivity experiences

These include ideas that thought or emotions are being externally controlled or that ideas are being withdrawn from, or inserted into, the mind.

2. Auditory hallucinations in the third person

These may be voices commenting on or discussing the thoughts or behaviour of the patient and are definitely perceived as being outside himself.

3. Primary delusions

Although these may arise from normal perceptions they give rise to beliefs which have no grounding in previous experience.

Having seized on some hard facts for a change, now refer your mind back to the experiential theories of schizophrenia expounded by Laing (1960) or to Szasz's doubts (1962) about the functions and validity of diagnosis. A student who finds the debate and ambiguities of psychiatry both boring and frustrating may be tempted to stick to something cut and dried, like amputations. But even then they may find that any branch of medicine contains its own dichotomies or irregularities simply because patients are people. Any individual whose social, intellectual, emotional and historical features were as predictable as his skeleton would not be particularly interesting to know anyway.

Social reactiveness

The ways in which disabilities associated with schizophrenia are affected by the social environment of the patients are of particular interest to occupational therapists.

Wing & Brown (1970) differentiate three types of impairment:

1. *Premorbid handicap*: Disabilities which are present before the overt onset of schizophrenia, such as a poor education, a difficult personality, a physical disability or low intelligence.

2. *Primary handicap*: Disabilities which are basically part of the illness, such as incoherent thought processes, delusional motivation or catatonic slowness or apathy.

3. *Secondary handicap*: Disabilities which are not part of the illness itself but which have accumulated because the patient has been ill, and because of his own and other people's reaction to the illness.

Primary handicaps may be further divided into two main groups. Florid symptoms, which are the features which normal people do not display, such as delusions, hallucinations, over-active or bizarre behaviour and incoherent expression of ideas. Defect symptoms relate to features lacking in the schizophrenic patient in comparisoin with a normal person; these include low levels of motivation and activity, social withdrawal, poverty of speech and thought and a lack of expressed emotion.

Secondary handicaps include the reaction of the individual to his own illness, which will depend upon the resources and integrity of his personality as well as upon the severity of his symptoms. The reaction of others to the sick person and to the degree of support that he requires will also affect the nature of his secondary handicap. Institutionalism, already discussed, is a special handicap belonging to this secondary group.

The social environment of the patient is deeply implicated in the degree and development of each of these types of handicap. In the case of the premorbid impairments the connection is obvious. The effect of the social environment on the florid and defect symptoms of primary handicap has been the subject of a number of studies (Wing & Freudenberg, 1961; Brown et al, 1962, 1966; Brown & Birley, 1968). In rather simplified terms an over-stimulating environment tends to lead to an exacerbation of florid symptoms, and an under-stimulating environment to a more gradual increase in defect symptoms. An over-stimulating environment can be created in hospital by a change in ward or programme, over-intense rehabilitation prior to discharge or to overactive and insensitive therapists or nurses. Outside hospital a similar problem can arise from the presence of over-intrusive close relatives or from an emotionally highly charged environment; such features tend to increase the likelihood of readmission to Hospital (Wing et al, 1964; Goldberg et al, 1977). On the other hand an impoverished social environment, typified by lengthy periods of inactivity, a regimented routine and possession of few private belongings or opportunities to make decisions, can have an equally damaging effect. Social withdrawal can deepen and the general negative effects of institutionalism increase.

This implies that an optimum environment needs to be created in order for the patient to maintain his health. Chapter 8 briefly describes the responsibilities of the therapist in this respect and also the necessity to enable the patient to monitor his own involvement in order to protect himself from the effects of under and overstimulation.

In the context of living within a family, Wing (1977) suggests the following list of provisions which are, to an extent, under the family's control:

1. Creating a non-critical, accepting environment
2. Providing the optimal degree of social stimulation
3. Keeping aims realistic
4. Learning to cope with fluctuating insight
5. Learning to respond to delusions and bizarre behaviour
6. Making use of whatever social and medical help is available
7. Learning to use welfare arrangements
8. Obtaining rewards from the patients presence
9. Helping patients' attitudes to self, to relatives, to medication, to work.

The majority of these factors are equally significant to an occupational therapist who is devising a programme of rehabilitation or designing an environment for treatment. It is important to realize that, just as we can improve a patient's condition, capabilities and confidence, we can also make him worse. There is a surprisingly narrow path to be beaten between increasing on one hand the patient's dependency and social withdrawal, and on the other making personal demands on him that he is unable to cope with.

Points of interest

The amount of research which has been carried out into the psychological and physiological features of the schizophrenic patient does not lend itself to simple summary. Parts of this research do, however, suggest that occupational therapists could be more specific in their work with these patients. The following selection of points of interest should suggest, to a practising occupational therapist, some promising lines of enquiry.

L. J. King (1974) described the typical physical posture and patterns of movement of a schizophrenic patient. These include an S-shaped posture from head to toe, a shuffling gait, flexed, adducted and internally rotated positioning of upper and lower limbs and a limited range of gross arm movement. In addition she noted immobility of the neck and shoulder girdle and a deficit in hand movements and grip. The use of physical exercise to improve these physical limitations appears also to affect the motivation and social interaction of the patients concerned. The suggested connection

is that schizophrenic patients may have deficits in proprio-
ceptive feedback. The kinetic sense or vestibular mechanisms are particularly implicated, a disturbance in this
modality reducing the patient's ability to integrate other
sensory information. If this is so, and if emphasis on movement and co-ordination within treatment can help to alleviate
perceptual and other problems associated with schizophrenia, then physical exercise which has for a long time
been included within treatment without profound theoretical
justification should gain both a new significance and more
specific application.

Schizophrenic patients are often very easily distracted and
find difficulty in processing sensory information in a meaningful way. They are also overinclusive in their use of
concepts, which means that they cannot always recognise the
boundaries between one idea or object and another. For
example they find it difficult to classify groups of objects or
to explain abstract ideas as expressed in proverbs. If a
person's thoughts are not being organised by consistent
relationships and by an appreciation of relevance then he can
tend to produce a flow of loosely connected ideas or words
with bizarre results.

Associations formed for the schizophrenic patient by
others, for example through praise, prompting or disapproval
can also be intrusive if not related to the task in hand.
External reinforcing cues will help him to organise his behaviour as long as he does not generalize to relate the affective
stimuli to a range of irrelevant activity.

The distractibility of patients can be related to problems of
awareness or arousal. It is possible that schizophrenic
patients may experience an abnormally high level of cortical
arousal, even though they may not be engaged in purposeful
activity. McGhie et al (1969) suggest that these patients may
suffer from a breakdown in the filter mechanism which
normally limits sensory input to a level at which the brain can
deal with it. Broen (1968) suggests, as an alternative, that
there is a ceiling on response strength which is particularly
low in schizophrenic patients. The presence of anxiety means
that this ceiling is reached even more quickly. The range of
possible responses to a situation may therefore all be at
'ceiling' or maximum strength, no particular alternative

dominating the others. This means, in simple terms, that the patient does not know what to do and is as likely to make an irrelevant response as an appropriate one.

Whatever the dynamics at cortical level, theories such as these suggest that a schizophrenic patient experiences a very chaotic world and may be bewildered by his own sensory input. These stimuli compete with each other for his attention and his responses are difficult to determine or to organize. Such a situation may explain not only bizarre behaviour or ideas but also the tendency to become socially withdrawn.

THE VULNERABLE PERSONALITY

The people whom we are trying to help are not all schizophrenic, dementing, intellectually impaired or otherwise neatly labelled within a medical frame of reference. They may have been given separate labels, it is true, such as 'inadequate personality', 'psychopath', 'chronic depressive', or 'paranoid', but they all have in common an inability to survive independently within society.

It is tempting to believe that, in pre-technological days, the weak and the eccentric were absorbed into the community and valued for what they could do. Alas, just as many schizophrenics must have been either canonised or burnt as witches, many other abnormal personalities must have suffered punishment or ridicule. Our present dilemma is a little more sophisticated and although we still vacillate between correcting those who do not adhere to the rules of society and offering nurture and support to those who cannot cope with it, the arguments on either side are supported by a good deal more theoretical ammunition.

Those who cannot operate within the society which we have constructed include a number of different 'types'. There is the agressive male who fails to learn, amongst other things, to love or to be loved. There is the timid man who has lost his mother and never managed to find a replacement. There is the adult who has too much invested in childhood to risk the responsibilities of a mature relationship. There is the gentle lady who nursed both parents through terminal illnesses but who now does not know who she is. There is the runt of the litter who, for complex family reasons, has been treated for decades for 'nerves'. Actually to cartoon these individuals as 'types' is just as bad as giving them diagnostic labels but it is difficult to find any other way to indicate their variety. Each, if unsupported, will tend either to exploit others or to be exploited. In hospital they are in danger of becoming too dependent on support or controls offered by staff. In the community the catastrophic nature of their lives can involve entraordinary numbers of professional staff, family members and others, all trying to unravel different parts of the puzzle. Whatever the circumstances of their treatment or care, a prior need is often for one of the people involved to act as a co-ordinator of others' efforts. He can then identify the main problems, the gaps in the service and the attempts at manipulation. It is, unfortunately, only too easy for the patient to become highly dependent on such a central figure and remain no nearer to the central goal of treatment, that of assuming responsibility for his own life.

THE MENTALLY HANDICAPPED

Mental handicap is not a psychiatric illness; these are two quite different things. The reason for including the mentally handicapped here is because so many of them experience long-term institutional care.

Mental handicap is the failure of intellectual development due to damage to the brain before, during or shortly after birth. Mental illness usually occurs later in life and is not normally attributable to retardation but may arise from a wide range of organic or social problems. An individual who is mentally handicapped may, of course, develop additional mental illness. Being mentally handicapped does not prevent one from becoming depressed, anxious, or from suffering from psychotic disorders. Because many mentally handicapped children are separated from their families and do not experience either a normal upbringing or the development of close personal relationships, they may be more vulnerable to additional emotional and behavioural problems.

Range of disability

Many attempts have been made to classify the mentally handicapped into discrete subgroupings. This has administrative advantages since different groups can be supposed to have different educational, organisational and protective needs. Classification also facilitates research and treatment based on scientific principles. Inevitably the classifications used by doctors, administrators, educators, legal specialist, supportive services and families are based on different criteria. For example the use of diagnostic criteria would divide patients into subgroups suffering from the effects of trauma, early infection, chromosomal abnormalities etc. Use of the intelligence quotient as a criterion could result in identifying those with an IQ of below 50, of between 50 and 70 and above 70. It is difficult to define criteria for classifying social competence and yet it is one of the concepts used within the British legal definitions of subnormality and severe subnormality. For the purposes of administration and research the mentally handicapped can be divided, for example, into those receiving or awaiting education in special schools, and those in hospital care, local authority care, attending training centres and/or living at home.

Although the severely handicapped can be identified fairly easily it is more difficult to find criteria for enumerating the mildly affected, so there is inevitably some dispute about how many mentally handicapped people there are within the population. Clarke & Clarke (1974) cite a figure of 2% but this may be low if one considers all those who are 'at risk' by not being able to cope within an industrial society due to intellectual impairment.

An occupational therapist may find it useful to think in terms of the following division, based on the problems the mentally handicapped present, rather than any diagnostic classification.

1. Those so acutely disabled as to need basic bedside care.
2. Severely handicapped people living either at home or in hospital who need basic training in communication and personal care.
3. Those who may have varying degrees of handicap but who

have produced secondary behavioural problems which require intervention.

4. Those who have the potential to live independent lives but who are at present receiving day or residential care during a period of training or preparation.
5. Semi-independent people either living in a hostel or attending sheltered workshops and who need continuing training and support.

Although all these groups are of interest and relevance, particular note should be made of the third, those with secondary behavioural problems. This is not an uncommon circumstance, arising from social situations, including institutions, and from the inability of patients with limited expressive vocabulary to indicate their frustrations in other ways. Professor Bicknell (1980) suggests that:

> Behavioural disturbance should no longer be seen as merely irritating, inconvenient and a reason for seeking a transfer to another set of caratakers but as a piece of non verbal communication signifying distress.

This would indicate that, although behavioural methods of treatment may be appropriate to correct maladaptive responses, it is equally important to try to interpret behaviour and to help the individual patient to find alternative ways of communicating his needs or his frustrations.

Specific problems

Copeland et al (1976) divide therapeutic concern into six important subjects:

1. Gross motor skills
2. Fine motor skills
3. Perceptual motor skills
4. Activities of daily living
5. Personal-social skills
6. Communication.

This seems to be a useful division since it relates to sequences of normal development and provides a framework for the assessment and treatment of a wide range of severe or mild handicaps.

Gross motor skills involve co-ordinated movement of the whole body such as in walking, running and jumping. Use of physical games, dancing and movement to music can be used to develop these skills.

Fine motor movements include precise manipulation of tools and more delicate movement of parts of the body.

Perceptual motor skills are more complex than the first two since they involve not only movement, but the processing of sensory information which motivates and directs that movement. The individual requires to integrate knowledge of his own physical orientation, through all of his senses, with knowledge of external objects. This involves an understanding of concepts such as behind, in front, left, right, above and below, as well as perceptual skills such as 'figure-ground discrimination'. The mentally handicapped person may be slow in processing and co-ordinating all this information in order to be able to perform tasks such as hitting a target, drawing, participating in ball games or just making sense of his environment.

Activities of daily living are generally described within Chapter 10. Mentally handicapped patients may experience problems in this due to perceptual-motor difficulties — to lack of fine motor skills as well as to lack of understanding or learning.

Personal and social skills involve the quality of interaction with other people and the range of roles that the patient is able to take. Although some of these skills relate to factors such as intelligence, concentration and motivation, it is equally important to consider the self-concept of the patient and the dynamics behind the construction of such an identity.

Communication is often a basic difficulty for mentally handicapped patients. Two important aspects are relevant to treatment. The first is the mode of communication, whether the patient needs to develop verbal vocabulary or whether a 'signing' system such as 'Makaton' needs to be employed. The second is the quality of communication, whether the patient is able to convey his needs and ideas without having recourse to disruptive behaviour or physical complaints in order to express difficulties or confusion.

The treatment of mentally handicapped children and adults is too specialized to be entirely embraced here. Although behavioural methods sometimes appear to be the most appropriate or most effective, this does not exclude the necessity to 'listen' to each patient's presentation of self and to be sensitive to expressions of need or individuality.

BIBLIOGRAPHY

Bicknell J 1980 Behavioural disturbance in the mentally handicapped person. Sandors Products, Middlesex
Broen W E 1968 Schizophrenia; research and theory. Academic Press, New York
Brown G W et al 1962 The influence of family life on the course of schizophrenic illness. British Journal of Preventative Social Medicine 16:55
Brown G W et al 1966 Schizophrenia and social care: a comparitive follow-up of 339 schizophrenic patients. Mandsley Monograph No 17; Oxford University Press, London
Brown G W, Birley J L T 1968 Crisis and life changes and the onset of schizophrenia. Journal of Health and Social Behaviour 9:203
Clare A 1976 Psychiatry in dissent. Tavistock, London
Clarke A M, Clarke A D B (eds) 1974 Mental deficiency the changing outlook. Methuen, London
Copeland M, Ford K, Solon N 1976 Occupational therapy for mentally retarded children. University Park Press, Baltimore
Goldberg et al 1977 Prediction of relapse in schizophrenic outpatients treated by drug and sociotherapy. Archives of General Psychiatry, London
King L J 1974 A sensory-integrative approach to schizophrenia. American Journal of Occupational Therapy 28:9: 529–536
McGhie A 1969 Pathology of attention. Penguin, Harmondsworth
Mittler P 1979 People not patients. Methuen, London
Savage R D, Britton P G, Bolton N, Hall E H 1973 Intellectual functioning in the aged. Methuen, London
Wing J K 1977 Schizophrenia and its management in the community. National Schizophrenia Fellowship, Surbiton
Wing et al 1964 Morbidity in the community of schizophrenic patients discharged from London mental hospitals in 1959. British Journal of Psychiatry 110:10
Wing J K, Freudenberg R K 1961 Social treatment of chronic schizophrenia: a comparative study of three mental hospitals. Journal of Mental Science 107:847
Wing J K, Brown G W 1970 Institutionalism and schizophrenia. Cambridge University Press, Cambridge
Wing J K, Morris B (eds) 1981 Handbook of psychiatric rehabilitation practice. Oxford University Press, Oxford

RECOMMENDED READING

Carver V, Liddiard P (eds) 1978 An aging population. Open University Press and Hodder and Stoughton, Sevenoaks

Coulter J 1973 Approaches to insanity. Pitman Press, Bath
Denham M J 1983 Care of the long-stay elderly patient. Croom Helm, London
Forrest A, Affleck J 1975 New perspectives in schizophrenia. Churchill Livingstone, Edinburgh
Gray B, Isaacs B 1979 Care of the elderly mentally infirm. Tavistock Publications, London
Innes W 1981 Psychiatry: a confused profession. Pupuke Press, Auckland
Pearce J M C 1984 Dementia. Blackwell, Oxford
Pitt B 1982 Psychogeriatrics. Churchill Livingstone, Edinburgh
Taylor D 1979 Schizophrenia? Office of Health Economics, London
Townsend J Marshall 1976 Self-concept and the institutionalization of mental patients: an overview and critique. Journal of Health and Social Behaviour 17: 263–271
Wendel W M 1976 Schizophrenia, the experience and its treatment. Jossey-Bass, San Fransisco

7

Assessment

REASONS FOR ASSESSMENT

Before it is possible to set specific goals for a patient, and to plan how he is to achieve these, it is necessary to know about his present abilities and situation. The process of assessment is one of collecting information systematically and organising it in a relevant and useful way.

It should be noted that assessing a patient's abilities does not in itself improve them. At the most it may enable him to form a more realistic view of his own progress and reassure him that some positive concern is being shown for his future. Assessment is a vital function of an occupational therapist but time invested in testing, measuring, plotting, filming and describing behaviour is wasted unless it is followed by some consequence. This may take the form of treatment or of placement in an optimum environment.

The major reasons for carrying out assessment prior to treatment are:

To give a clear description of his present limitations

Such limitations may be due to his normal abilities being overridden by the symptoms or consequences of illness. They may be due to the effects of his social environment or of institutional living. They may be due to a failure to develop skills during a period in life when they are normally acquired. Because any one or any combination of these factors may be responsible, the therapist should be aware of the patient's medical and personal history.

To indicate the patient's assets

Very few people have a completely balanced range of skills. Most have an interesting pattern of strengths, weaknesses and mediocrities which has evolved from individual interests and opportunities for experience. It can be a mistake to assign all a patient's apparent inabilities or areas of confusion to his status as a sick person. There is, after all, no case for admitting every occupational therapy student who cannot make pastry to a psychiatric hospital. It is equally important to recognise a patient's particular aptitudes or abilities; these may give indications of his potential ability in other areas or may have relevance to plans for his resettlement and future lifestyle.

To establish a baseline for treatment

This is closely connected with the first reason given but the word 'baseline' requires emphasis since this is the point from which treatment can be planned and against which improvement can be compared. The description of behaviour therefore has to be constructed in such a way that later comparisons can be made.

To assign a patient to an appropriate group

A great deal of treatment is carried out in groups rather than purely on a one-to-one sessional basis. This does not preclude the use of individual plans for treatment but does involve, for each patient, the selection of appropriate companions. Some groups may be assembled on the basis of common need, for example a domestic group comprising those for whom the learning of domestic tasks is a priority; a 'communication group' for those who have particular problems in formulating and expressing ideas; a 'pre-work group', a 'social skills group' or a 'personal care group'. Other groups are formed on the basis of the more general level of ability of each of its members. The group stays together for a wide range of activities and movement from one group to another is made according to progress in combination of skills or functions.

The major reasons for subsequent assessment are:

For comparison with previous results

The two questions which should concern a therapist are whether the patient is benefiting by becoming more skilled, happier or more confidfent and whether the treatment being offered is appropriate and of good quality. When the results of assessments made over a period of time are compared with each other there are three possible results: these are 'deterioration', 'no change' or 'improvement'. Deterioration could be due to a worsening of the patient's clinical condition or social situation or could indicate that the treatment he is receiving is a load of rubbish. 'No change' may be, in a deteriorating condition, a victory. It could equally well be a reflection of inadequate treatment or could imply that the patient is already functioning at his maximum potential. Improvement may be appropriate and well managed, but it could also be unrelated to the intervention of the occupational therapist.

This may sound complicated or depressing but it need not necessarily be so. Essentially, it is not good enough to compare the results of a series of assessments and use them to label the patient as good, bad or indifferent. The consequences are more far reaching and should be used to make intelligent suggestions about relevant causes and effects. The mechanics of assessment are much easier than the sensitive interpretation of results.

To plan subsequent stages of treatment

The first plan that was made, or the first goals which were set, may prove to have been short-sighted, inadequate or over-ambitious. This is natural; the only wrong decision, in general terms, is not to make any future decisions or amendments. Long-term patients often require long-term plans that are sequential but require constant re-evaluation in order to get the timing right or to embrace current problems.

To make recommendations for the future

When a patient is due to make a change from the regime of care that he has been receiving it is important that he moves into a living or working environment which will maintain his health. Some of the possible environments are briefly described in Chapters 9 and 10. An informed and appropriate recommendation at this stage, which takes into account capability, tolerance to stress and the patient's own desires, may help to prevent future distress or admission.

These general reasons for assessment relate mainly to the patient but there are two other factors which need to be examined and evaluated within treatment. The first is the activity which the patient is to be engaged in. Activities can only be used as a form of treatment if the therapist is aware of the precise demands and skills which they involve. The process of studying an activity and breaking it down into its component parts is known as 'activity analysis' or 'task analysis'. A framework for doing this is suggested in Chapter 11.

The second factor is the environment and the skills which the patient will require in the future in order to be able to cope. This future environment may include sheltered work, a new place to live, a different group of people to relate to, or complete independence. The therapist cannot control the future environment but should be able to make predictions about the benefits or stresses which it may create. This is why it is important to study the abilities and qualities of those who are coping successfully in any environment which has been proposed for the future of a patient. It is also important to recognise the factors in the environment which most frequently contribute to breakdown or readmission.

A GLOBAL VIEW

Assessment is not something which occurs only on admission

or prior to discharge as a separate process from the rest of the programme. Knowledge about a patient's abilities or difficulties not only enables the therapist to embark on planning but also provides a continuous flow of information about the patient's progress and the suitability of the programme.

Before thinking in detail about specific areas of assessment, or about selecting an approach to treatment, it can be useful to stand back and consider this simple A, B, C.

Attributes and *attitudes* are the patient's personal starting point. Under these headings can be included his level of intellectual functioning, his perception of himself and others, his emotional bonds, personality traits, motivation and current strategies for coping.

Barriers and *battles* are the factors which prevent him from fulfilling a satisfying and autonomous role within society. These may be symptoms or consequences of illness, may arise from his social situation, may include physical handicaps or relate to lack of opportunity.

Capabilities and *choices* are the things that he is able to do. These may be work, social or personal skills which have been acquired through treatment or which have been preserved despite illness. Choice is important since he is more likely to extend skills which relate to his personal enjoyment or satisfaction and which are relevant to the life style which he would like to adopt.

It must be quite apparent that there is a great deal of overlap between these three headings. They are not offered as a checklist of functions but aim to provide a more complete view of any patient's total situation. It is necessary to think in broad concepts, such as this, before fragmenting one's concerns into the smaller, practical issues such as handling money, boiling eggs, greeting strangers and cutting toe nails. The therapist who fails to perceive an individual as a three-dimensional and complex pattern tends to end up with a list of tasks which he can or cannot do. This in turn leads to a corrective style of treatment which aims to patch up deficits piecemeal rather than to develop potential.

THE BASIC METHODS

When it comes to 'how' to assess there are five basic methods which again may overlap with each other or be combined. These are observation, interview, self-rating, standardized tests and performance checks.

Observation

Observing others is one of the commonest activities in the world. Most people observe in an unstructured way, failing to distinguish between information, impression and the effects of personal bias. To use observation as a tool for assessment it is necessary to select relevant material and organise personal perceptions in an ordered manner. A patient should be observed in a number of different settings whilst engaged in a range of tasks in order to gain a more comprehensive picture.

There are a lot of questions which you can ask yourself about another person, for example:

Personal appearance. Is the individual neat or untidy? If his clothes are his own what styles or colours does he choose? How concerned is he about cleanliness or personal grooming?

Posture and movement. How does he stand or walk or sit? Are his movements purposeful or vague? How does he hold his head? Is he well co-ordinated or clumsy?

Manner. Does he appear relaxed and at ease? Does he look tense or uncomfortable? Does he give the impression of being subservient, socially equal or superior to others, and exactly how is this impression conveyed?

Facial expression. Does he make appropriate contact with his eyes or is his gaze too constant or averted? Does he smile or laugh and if so what triggers this response? Does he use his face to convey interest, disagreement, concurrence, boredom or distress? What is his habitual expression in respose? Incidentally, what is your habitual expression or are you unaware of it?

General level of activity. Does he fidget, make repetitive movements, chain smoke, keep touching himself, or find comfort in rubbing or rocking himself? Does he appear over-meticulous? Is he slow or lethargic?

Intentional activity. Does he spontaneously engage in activty and for how long? What starts him or stops him? How does he handle implements or materials? Does he use initiative or look to others for help?

Cognitive ability. Does he familiarize himself with new surroundings? Can he follow instructions? Does he remember what he is doing? Does his attention wander? Does he organize himself in relation to a task?

Communication. Does he place himself near other people? Does he initiate conversation? Does he direct or show concern for other people? How does he use his vocabulary? Does the content of his speech make sense? What is the tone and volume of his voice? Does he use non verbal forms of communication?

This list could go on much longer but the point should have been made by now that an enormous amount of information becomes available as soon as someone walks into a room. Problems arise when either we do not see it or we use it incorrectly.

Observation involves two major skills — being aware of information and avoiding its misinterpretation. The first can be acquired by practice, concentration and by the use of observation checklists which prompt one's attention to detail. Interpretation or the drawing of inferences can be severely affected by the observer's own expectations or perceptual and cognitive set. We all tend to take short cuts by perceiving a stranger as belonging to a general type, or having particular attributes on the flimsiest evidence. We warm to people, or take an instant dislike to them, for the most superficial reasons such as the colour of their hair, their name or their slight resemblance to someone else. If we are told that an individual is confused, depressed or deluded before meeting him we tend to be more sensitive towards evidence which will bear this out. It is also tempting to make assumptions or jump to conclusions about a person's mood or problems. Is the woman who stands weeping in the kitchen depressed, bereaved, angry or has she just jammed her thumb in the cutlery drawer? In fact we cannot know the meaning of what we observe without seeking further information to support or to discredit what is simply an impression. Observation only allows one to describe and infer.

Reliability arises not only from learning to observe patients more keenly but also from learning to observe and monitor one's own personal biases and habits of perception. It is also wise to compare the fruits of one's own observation with those of other people who have had similar opportunities.

A rather different and more structured way to use observation is to undertake 'activity sampling'. The individual is observed at fixed intervals, for example during 5 minutes every half hour or once every 3 minutes. The activity which is taking place is recorded on a rating scale or tally sheet. The most usual method of recording is to provide a series of alternatives which the observer can select and mark. At the end of the period of observation, which may be several days, the marks can be totalled giving a profile which shows the frequency and duration of each behaviour. The alternatives could include, for example:

Inactive and alone
Inactive in company
Talking to staff
Talking to peers
Solitary activity
Co-operative activity.

The design of each record sheet should be pertinent to the situation in which it is to be used. Observers need to be in agreement about the exact interpretation of each description if the study is to be reliable. Not only does this give an objective measure of baseline behaviour but one which can be readily compared at later stages of treatment.

This method of assessment was referred to within Chapter 1 and is particularly associated with behavioural approaches to treatment.

Interviews

An interview is a meeting between therapist and patient which takes place for a specific purpose. If it is arranged prior to planning treatment it is usually helpful if the therapist has already met the patient informally.

Most therapists have three major purposes during an interview; to gain information about the patient, to initiate or develop a relationship with him, and to explain the purpose of occupational therapy in the context of his own problems or participation. The interview also offers an opportunity to extend and explore inferences drawn from previous observations.

An interview must be planned carefully in terms of its environment, time and objectives. A relaxed atmosphere which is free from interruption, preferably in a place which is familiar to the patient, may be most helpful. Time should be allocated so that the patient is neither left hanging about nor made to feel that the therapist is preoccupied with other concerns or in a hurry to get away. The therapist should be clear about exactly what information is to be exchanged and why. There is a dichotomy of views as to whether one should study case notes prior to a first interview or not. If one does there is a danger of being influenced by diagnostic labelling and reports of previous behaviour. If one does not it is more difficult to formulate relevant lines of enquiry. Although an interview should have a clear structure the therapist may choose to use open-ended questions and encourage the patient to express ideas about his own situation, treatment and future. Listening involves giving one's entire attention to what someone else is saying instead of using their speaking time to decide what you are going to say next. Real listening requires great concentration and discipline, and is surprisingly difficult.

Information or impressions which can be gained from an interview include the patient's self-concept and attitude to both his condition and his treatment. It should be possible to gauge his degree of motivation and the extent to which he is able to plan for the future. Factual information can be obtained about his social history, previous work and leisure interests, current relationships and capabilities. Some patients become understandably fed up with being asked the same questions by a host of different people, so one should create a balance between demonstrating a genuine degree of interest and requesting information which can be easily obtained elsewhere. The worst interviews are conducted by therapists who use the situation to boost their own self-esteem.

During later stages of the interview the patient should be involved as much as possible in formulating the objectives and plans for his own treatment. He should know, even in simple terms, why he should do whatever he is intended to do. Information about occupational therapy in general should be kept brief and relevant to his own involvement. This is not a selling job, he will already have received from other patients and staff a crude evaluation of the department and its effectiveness. The only proof lies in his own eventual benefit. On the other hand enough information should be given to motivate his own attendance and participation.

The nature of the therapeutic relationship is extremely important at this stage. If you have not read Chapters 2 and 3 previously, this would be a good moment to do so.

Self-rating

This is a method of assessment normally associated with patients who are articulate and insightful. However it does have applications within long-term psychiatry.

'Self-rating' can be used to measure attitudes or to measure an individual's perception of his own performance. To ask someone to provide information about themselves in this way does raise problems of subjectivity and inaccuracy due to variations in mood, in desire to please or to confound the therapist or in lack of experience in using forms. On the other hand, the way in which a patient rates himself should be significant to the therapist and should also allow the patient to be more fully involved in the obejctives and progression of his own treatment. This can also be a tool for gradually altering the way in which he perceives himself in relation to other people.

The measurement of attitudes is partly attempted during interviews by the use of questionnaires, rating scales and written descriptions of events.

Questionnaires can be used to explore preferences for activity, perceptions of treatment or degrees of difficulty experienced. A variety of possible formats is shown in Figure 7.1. This is not exhaustive; the design of questionnaires is beyond the scope of this book, but the basic rules are:

1. Be clear about what information is to be obtained and why.
2. Choose a format which will be most easily understood.
3. Construct the questions avoiding unnecessary words or ambiguities.

4. Try it out on a sample of its intended respondents to see if it can be administered easily and if the results can be processed in a meaningful way.

1. Tick the activity which you like best: Gardening
   Quizzes
   Cooking
   Drama

2. Draw a circle round the word which best describes how you feel during the drama sessions:
   Enthusiastic. Happy. Positive. Apathetic. Resentful. Nervous.

3.	Agree	Disagree	Uncertain
i) Patients should only attend O. T. when they feel like it.			
ii) It is easy to get into conversation with other people.			

4. I found the following tasks:	Very easy	Easy	OK	Hard	Very hard
Following the recipe					
Weighing out the ingredients					
Choosing the best utensils etc.					

Figure 7.1 Styles of questionnaire

Rating scales can be used to find out how someone feels about his environment, his fellow patients, staff and activity. The two most usual forms are point scales and semantic differentials, both of which are described later in this chapter. Pairs of adjectives such as warm/cold, enthusiastic/apathetic, fair/unfair, worthless/valuable or tense/relaxed may be offered in relation to people, situations or events.

The individual's perception of his own performance may play a significant part in the running of a domestic training programme or of industrial therapy. To use the latter example, the patient's rating of his own work during a week may be used, in co-ordination with the therapist, to determine his rate of pay or bonuses.

Standardized tests

A standardized test is one which has been carefully researched for validity and reliability, which is comparable with established norms and which is administered by those specifically instructed in its use. Many occupational therapy schools use standardized tests of cognitive ability as part of their procedure for selecting students.

The easiest example to give of standardized tests in practical applications is a battery of assessments of working abilities. Patients may spend an extended period of assessment working through tests for filing ability, calculation, co-ordination between hand and eye, the use of written instruction, speed of performance or any other function which lends itself to objective measurement. Performance checks upon domestic and personal independence may also become standardized in use if they are able to stand up to rigorous testing. Many occupational therapy departments currently use assessment tests which have not been standardized. This does not necessarily mean that they are totally invalid or unreliable but they need to be applied with more caution, and time needs to be spent on studying and improving them so that they may become even more useful.

A revision of the implications of validity and reliability is provided later in this chapter under the heading 'The mechanics of assessment'. Here, however are the basic rules for standardizing a test:

1. Decide what function is to be tested.
2. Identify a task or format which relies on this function for successful completion. This is your independent variable.
3. List the factors which may be present as extraneous variables. These may include other skills which the patient may bring to bear on the task or may arise from the environment.
4. Eliminate as many of these extraneous variables as possible by devising written instructions for the administration of the test and the conditions under which it should be used.
5. Make a written record of variables which cannot be eliminated.
6. Devise a scoring or rating system which is easily understood and which does not lend itself to ambiguous or loose interpretation on the part of the tester.

7. Note that the score obtained by the subject is the dependent variable.

8. Try out the test using as many testers and subjects as possible. If the test is used twice on the same subject a difference in score may be due to difference between testers, to the effect of practice on the subject or the inevitable variations from test to test.

9. Adjust the task or the instructions until the scores given in a wide range of trials differ only within the limits recognised as having no statistical significance. This does involve acquiring a basic understanding of tests which can be used to indicate statistical significance. This is not impossible since statistics, like many other phenomena, relies more on mystique than complexity for its ability to terrify. But neverthelesss a tame mathematician or statistician can be an essential friend.

It is also possible to standardize less formal methods of assessment such as observation. Most ambiguities arise over the way in which information is described or recorded. Very briefly the steps towards standardizing an assessment form are as follows:

1. Design the form, possibly on one of the basic models given later in this chapter.

2. Provide a written explanation of its interpretation and use.

3. Use it for a while to familiarize staff with its format and to identify and correct any reported problems.

4. Carry out tests of reliability, either by involving several independent recorders in each assessment or by recording a patient's performance on film and asking a wide sample of observers to use the form in relation to that performance.

5. Keep adjusting it until it is proved to be reliable as above.

Performance checks

These are the widely used procedures for discovering and recording what a patient can actually do. The record should always be based on a demonstration of skills and not on the therapist's assumptions or the patient's assurances.

There is an endless range of abilities which may need to be assessed in this way. If you recorded in detail every task personally performed within the last week, the resulting check list could be longer than this book. To reduce the chaos of such a list it would have to be arranged under headings or areas of responsibility. The list can further be reduced by recognizing that capability in performing one task is reasonable evidence of being able to cope with a number of other tasks of similar complexity.

A great many check-lists exist and although it would seem more convenient to reduce the number to a few commonly used varieties, there are good reasons for so many having separately evolved. Firstly there is considerable variety in the skills which will be needed by patients destined to live in different settings. A performance check should relate closely to future needs. Secondly the extent to which each task needs to be broken down into its component parts for assessment depends on the levels of ability of the patients being assessed. To take a classic, and rather boring, example of cleaning teeth, in one unit the following breakdown of sequential tasks may be required with the possibility of rating degrees of independence in each separate stage:

1. Selects toothbrush
2. Turns tap on
3. Wets brush
4. Removes cap from toothpaste
5. Squeezes out correct amount on to brush
6. Brushes teeth — top, bottom, front, back
7. Rinses mouth
8. Rinses and replaces brush
9. Replaces cap on toothpaste
10. Cleans basin
11. Dries hands and mouth.

A form devised for a different group of patients may require a yes/no answer to the question 'Does he clean his teeth?' A third group of patients may have no teeth.

When a wide range of detail needs to be included within a performance check, separate records are normally made under a series of headings such as cognitive skills, motor skills, communication, personal care, domestic tasks, personal organization, safety and so on. A summary chart showing the relationship between different areas of ability can then be used.

THE MECHANICS OF ASSESSMENT

The basic assessment tools described above each contain different proportions of objectivity and subjectivity in application. An objective measurement is one which can be demonstrated to be both valid and reliable. It is easier to be objective in relation to a specific task such as wiring a plug, counting components or boiling an egg for $3\frac{1}{2}$ minutes. Other attributes are difficult to measure with the same precision but rely to a greater extent on the skills, discretion and experience of the therapist. These subjective areas include the ability, for example, to establish and maintain social contacts, to exercise initiative and to resolve domestic and other problems.

Where subjectivity is inevitable it should be recognised and if possible compensated for. Where objectivity is to be established certain concepts and strategies exist which assist towards accurate measurement and recording.

Validity, reliability and normative values

Validity refers to the extent to which a procedure tests what it sets out to test. For example, a valid test for accuracy of co-ordination between hand and eye should not be influenced by other factors such as speed, tolerance to noise or standing, hearing or intake of alcohol. To use an extreme example, I could not know anything about your ability to perform precise movements by asking you to thread a needle in the middle of a discotheque session after you have consumed half a bottle of wine on an empty stomach and lost one contact lens.

To test one element of performance without the results being confused by other skills or events is a matter of controlling the variables.

The independent variable is mainly within the tester's control. This is the situation which has been contrived in order to create the test. If you devise a speed test which involves inserting a number of pegs into a peg board, then factors such as the sizes of the pegs and board, and their relative starting positions, are included within your independent variables.

The dependent variable is what happens or, more correctly, is one factor inevitably linked to another, for example the number of pegs finally placed on the board. This, whatever the test, is the factor which one should be able to measure in order to compare the result with the performance of other people or to establish statistical averages or ranges or difference.

Extraneous variables are the things which can get in the way. These may be skills other than the one being assessed such as eyesight, comprehension of instructions or concentration. Equally they may be environmental influences such as the time of day, states of hunger, intergallactic war, lighting and seating or outside distractions. A large number of extraneous variables can be controlled by simple strategies such as keeping testing conditions constant, using specified instructions, and always checking that the subjects have their usual spectacles or hearing aids. Those variables that cannot be eliminated must at least be recognized.

Reliability means that the results of a test should be accurate and not dependent on variations of criteria between testers. If a test is reliable it should not matter who administers it providing that they adhere to the instructions. The score may be interpreted in the light of experience but the way in which that score is calculated should be constant. An example of an unreliable test is a point scale using such identifications as 'excellent', 'good', 'adequate', 'poor', and 'bad'. This would be dependent on an individual's interpretation of the scale and one therapist could habitually score higher or lower than another.

Normative values are a way of providing a comparative measure. If a large enough group of mathematics graduates completed a test in logic then the distribution of scores would give a 'norm' for mathematics graduates performing that task. A less group-specific norm could be obtained by applying the same test to a properly randomized sample of the general population. If you want to know the normative value of work skills within a specific sheltered workshop, then you will need to carry out tests on a number of people already working successfully within this environment. The obvious advantage of establishing norms of performance for different tasks is that when subsequently testing an individual the results acquire both relevance and meaning.

Methods of recording

The way in which an assessment is made is closely linked with the way in which it is recorded.

Some of the more usual forms are described below. Reasons for selecting one in preference to another should always be identified.

Point scales

Each skill or function is rated on a fixed scale. Each point on the scale may bear a number or a symbol but an explanation of criteria should be provided for interpretation. The simplest version would be a two point scale where the tester has a single choice between indicating that a patient *can* or *cannot* perform a task unaided. In a scale with more points a wider choice may be provided, for example *'Unable/able with assistance/able with verbal prompting/independent'*. The commonly used five point scale allows for a midway grading which can indicate average performance, whatever that means. The larger the number of points on a scale the more difficult it becomes for it to be used reliably.

This type of assessment form is useful for performance checks of domestic or personal activities such as cooking, washing, handling money and routine organisation. Its advantage lies in simplicity and ease of reference. The form does however need to be carefully worded and deisgned if it is to be useful.

Semantic differential

This type of record is designed so that two extremes of behaviour or of emotional response are represented at opposite sides.

MUTE _____ VERBOSE

TOTALLY _____ INITIATES
PASSIVE   ACTIVITY

or

WARM _____ COLD

WORTHLESS _____ VALUABLE

Figure 7.2 Semantic differential

It is proper to randomize positive and negative descriptions on either side of the page to counteract the effects of general bias.

The midline between the two extremes is marked. There are two basic ways of using such a system.

1. Columns are drawn, creating a series of boxes, which are headed, for example, 'definitely a, inclines to a, inclines to b, definitely b'. The boxes are ticked according to the perceptions of the assesor or of the patient if it is being used for self-rating.

2. The user makes a point anywhere between the two extremes without the aid of columns. This demands more comparative visual or special judgement but can be more flexible in areas where a degree of subjectivity has been accepted as being inevitable. Marks may be joined by a vertical line down the page, often resulting in a zigzag, which gives a visual profile of performance or attitudes. By comparing results, at different stages of treatment, changes can be seen.

Multiple choice statements

In this form the assessor is provided with a limited choice of statements. The statement under each heading which most closely approximates to the patient's observed behaviour is selected and marked.
For example:

Concentration
   a. Attention fleeting — needs prompting to continue task, attends to distractions at random, frequent errors
   b. Intermittent distraction — maintains attention for 5–10 minutes, some errors and need for prompting

    c. Concentrates well — only distracted by new stimuli, makes few or no errors due to inattention, needs no prompting

or

Timekeeping
    a. No concept of time
    b. Dependent on others for reminder
    c. Aware of time but habitually unreliable
    d. Occasionally late
    e. Consistently reliable in timekeeping.

Multiple choice statements have an advantage over point scales in that each alternative can be specifically worded under each item. Reliability is still dependent, however, on agreement between users about the exact interpretation of each alternative.

Charts and diagrams

These strategies allow a summary of the patient's abilities to be represented in diagrammatical form for immediate reference. The Gunzberg Progress Assessment Charts form a useful example. Under part of this system information is recorded by shading in appropriately numbered boxes within a segmented circle. White areas on the chart indicate skills which are lacking. A detailed key and instruction manual are required in order to maintain reliability.

It is not difficult to represent a range of information diagrammatically or even pictorially. The purpose of doing so is partly for speed of reference for members of staff. Of equal importance though is the possibility of making this information both meaningful and available to the patient. Even the recording of assessments can be used to involve an individual in his own treatment.

Reporting

One of the consequences of having carried out the assessment of a patient is the ability to submit a useful report to other members of the team. The record of assessment is, in itself, seldom applicable. What is required by others is a summary and interpretation of what has been taking place within the occupational therapy department, together with plans for further treatment or recommendations for the future. Most colleagues appreciate reports which are brief and relevant but that indicate the availability of further information if it is required. Correct use of medical terminology is helpful in order to keep communication concise and accurate but this should not be extended to the use of professional jargon. A well presented description in good English is actually far more impressive than a jumble of words which are too long and abbreviations which are too short.

Some reports are submitted for specific reasons related to discharge or referral and their contents cannot be predicted here. General progress reports can, however, be more standardised in content and could answer all or or some of the following questions:

1. What implications have arisen from assessment of the patient's ability or progress?
2. What problem or problems have been identified as being particularly relevant to occupational therapy?
3. What are the current aims of treatment and what immediate goals have been set?
4. What programme of treatment has been designed for the patient and for how long will this be in force?
5. What assistance or co-operation, from other members of the team, would be appreciated by the occupational therapy department?
6. What help or information can the occupational therapy department provide for others in respect of this patient?
7. Any other difficulties experienced, successes to be noted or recommendations to be made?

Within occupational therapy departments, and in a broader context in some hospitals, reporting consists of less formal, verbal communication. Although verbal reporting sounds easier, many people find it to be more difficult than the provision of written material. This is not really surprising since, when giving a written report, there is more time to think and less temptation to be purely anecdotal. Verbal reporting is an important part of every day in a busy department and can stimulate new ideas or a new direction of treatment. It is different from written reporting in that it can be more immediate, more frequent and sometimes more creative. Verbal reporting alone, however, can cause stagnation or a casual attitude towards the problems experienced by patients. There is a discipline in having to write down what is known and what is intended which can be helpful not only to the team but to the occupational therapist. The most effective system of reporting is likely to be a combination of verbal discussion and written plans or recommendations.

RECOMMENDED READING

Clarke D H 1981 Social therapy in psychiatry, 2nd edn. Churchill Livingstone, Edinburgh

Cook M 1979 Perceiving others. Methuen, London

Henerson M E, Lyons Morris L, Taylor Fitz-Gibbon C 1978 How to measure attitudes. Sage Publications, Beverly Hills

Hopkins H L, Smith H D 1978 Willard and Spackman's occupational therapy, 5th edn. Lippincott, New York

Kahn R L, Cannell C F 1957 The dynamics of interviewing. John Wiley, New York

Lyons Morris L, Taylor Fitz-Gibbon C 1978 How to measure achievement. Sage Publications, Beverly Hills

Mittler P 1979 People not patients. Methuen, London

Mosey A C 1970 Three frames of reference for mental health. Charles B. Slack, New Jersey

Oppenheim A N 1966 Questionnaire design and attitude measurement. Heinemann, London

Reed K, Sanderson S R 1980 Concepts of occupational therapy. William and Wilkins, Baltimore

Wing J K, Morris B (eds) 1981 Handbook of psychiatric rehabilitation practice. Oxford University Press, Oxford

8

The design of treatment

The last chapter considered some of the ideas and methods involved in assessment. Earlier chapters introduced clinical problems and the different theoretical standpoints from which such problems are perceived and treated. It now becomes necessary to discuss what to do with all this knowledge or information so that it may become relevant to the practical problems of an individual patient. This will involve the organisation of information and the process of setting goals, planning programmes and monitoring results.

THE ORGANISATION OF INFORMATION

Relevant knowledge

In order to plan the treatment of any patient an occupational therapist needs to integrate a wide range of information from a variety of sources. This information will include, although not necessarily in this order of importance, the following:

1. Knowledge of the patient's clinical condition if diagnosed, the treatment he is receiving from other members of the team and its possible results.

2. The theoretical, concepts on which treatment may be based and the reasons for selecting or combining these.

131

3. The clinical history of the patient, whether his problems are long standing, cyclical, intermittent, degenerative, related to stress or to long term dependence, and what therapies have been used previously and with what effect.

4. The social background and history including important relationships, both in the past and still existing, personal trauma, employment, interests and the existence of future support or future social stresses.

5. The results of assessment of ability in cognitive areas, communication and relationships, personal care, working skills and any other test or evaluation carried out.

6. The likely time available for treatment, having regard to the duration of admission to hospital or to day-care unit, the therapist's time, aspects of the patient's routine and any other constraints.

7. The most likely future needs of the patient.

There is no point in obtaining this plethora of information unless you can do something with it. The first thing to do is to reduce it to a manageable size. The detailed knowledge of his condition and his personal history may not all be relevant to his present problems. With some experience the therapist should be able to select pertinent factors against which the rest becomes background. Background features can always be brought into focus again if something occurs which draws attention to them. A pertinent factor is one which appears to have a direct bearing on the patient's current concerns or behaviours.

It may be unrealistic to believe that all the patient's difficulties can be resolved through occupational therapy. Such a belief may lead to a programme which is too diverse to be effective.

From the raw information suggested above the therapist needs to:

Identify problems

These should not be generalized features such as that the patient is depressed, withdrawn, confused, excited or irrational. In fact it is better not to think in symptomatic terms. It is a problem, for example, if he is unable to plan aspects of his own activity, if he cannot maintain a conversation, get on with his neighbours, look after his own personal needs or complete simple tasks. The more specifically problems can be identified the easier it becomes to set relevant objectives. The whole treatment team, including the patient, should be involved in making this identification.

Establish priorities

Several factors have to be balanced here. Many abilities can be sequentially learned, one level being attained before the next is attempted. Tackling one problem, such as a poor concentration span may result in improvement in other problems. The patient's perception of the most important problems may differ from that of the staff. If his current concerns or wishes are ignored, his attitude towards treatment may naturally be affected.

Select the area of intervention

It is better to do the thing that you are good at well than to try to muscle in on other people's skills. It is quite possible that psychiatrists, psychologists, nurses, social workers, link-therapists and physiotherapists, as well as occupational therapists, will all get to heaven. But only if they communicate, co-operate and agree mutual strategies and individual areas of responsibility. The problem or problems on which the occupational therapist is going to concentrate should be selected, defined and known by others.

The complexity of organising information, and extracting from it factors relevant to a defined hierarchy of problems, is the reason why students of occupational therapy and other disciplines are required to produce case studies. Because it is difficult it needs to be practised and the results presented in such a way that teachers and peers can offer constructive criticism or support. The discipline of having to record detailed case studies which demonstrate the reasoning behind treatment should not, of course, be reserved for students. As a regular feature of professional work this process enables therapists to gain confidence and improvement in clinical skills, to direct their own continuing study, to teach more clearly and to add to available professional literature. It is a fallacy that an unusual or atypical patient is the best subject for a detailed case study. You may not meet another one. It is the treatment currently being offered to large numbers of people which most needs re-examination and research.

Progressive patterns

In Chapter 5 the use of models, which may lend themselves to diagrammatical representation, was mentioned. A simplified version of the following structure, Figure 8.1, was used as an example.

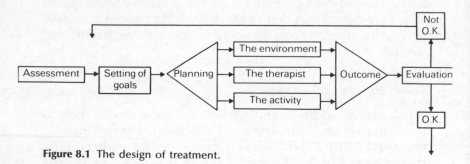

Figure 8.1 The design of treatment.

With this chapter we have arrived near the middle of this diagram. It is a relatively straightforward representation of the process of treatment showing the order in which stages are normally considered.

There are in existence far more complex models showing the wide spectrum of human activity which should be considered within treatment. There are many ways of representing the different stages of treatment, and the decisions to be made at each, the different outcomes and the future strategies. Diagrams proposed within current professional literature include concentric circles, boxes, charts, spirals or landscapes of converging arrows.

One of the immediate virtues of a tidy diagram is that it makes the therapist feel better. This is, of course, a good thing, but it is also useful to have a sequential guide to practice or a checklist of factors to be considered and comprehended before planning treatment. A structured concept of the entire process facilitates teaching, research and a critical approach to the therapy currently being offered. Some of the most effective charts or diagrams are those drawn up by individual therapists in order to clarify and structure their own thoughts.

On the other hand the problems of an individual cannot always be resolved by geometry or semantics. It is dangerous to adhere rigidly to one perception of treatment to the extent that it blunts the edge of creative or independent thought.

To return to the model to which we are loosely adhering the next stages are the setting of goals and the planning of programmes. Beyond these are a triptych of boxes representing the tools of environment, activity and therapist. The first two of these are each expanded in a separate chapter. The therapist is as much a constant theme as the patient and an understanding of this role should be extracted from the whole.

STATING INTENTIONS

There are at least three good reasons for stating what you are intending to do before you do it.

1. It allows clearer planning of the use of time and activity and enables the therapist to evaluate the effectiveness of treatment. If you know where you are going then, relatively, you know where you are.

2. It allows those to whom we are accountable to understand our actions and recognise both achievements and problems. These people include medical colleagues, patients and members of the general public.

3. It enables others to co-operate with us. Patients, and colleagues who are equally concerned in their care, need to know the purpose of any programme and the results that are hoped for.

Aims, goals and objectives

These are all familiar terms but confusion sometimes arises about how to discriminate between them.

An aim is a statement of the general condition which one hopes to achieve. A student may aim to become an occupational therapist. An occupational therapist may aim to improve the communication skills of a group of patients. Patients may aim to lead a life independent of medical care. An aim need not be expressed in precise behavioural terms but is used to indicate the direction of movement. An aim can be stated using comfortably vague verbs such as 'improve', 'develop' and 'experience'. It can include abstract concepts such as being happier, feeling more confident, expressing feelings and making friends. An aim can also relate to a future environment or status such as working in open employment, being discharged to a group home, being happily married or being independent in personal care. In some literature the term 'end-goal' is used in a very similar fashion.

A goal should be a much precise statement of intended activities and results. It may relate to a very limited but specific activity such as washing, using a telephone, cooking a meal, attending a meeting or staying sober for one day. Because even simple goals may need to be broken down into a number of different skills or processes they need to be set individually, in relation to the needs and capabilities of each patient. Where many stages are involved these can be referred to as subgoals. Essentially goals are constructed to form realistic and measurable targets on the way towards fulfilling an aim. They are simple in that they relate to a precise activity or achievement but need careful construction if they are to be useful. For this reason the next two sections are devoted to formulating goals for patients and for staff. The interpretation of the word 'goal' used subsequently covers the terms 'sub-goals' 'intermediate objectives' and 'steps' which may be encountered elsewhere.

An objective, or more properly an object, is a term which has become popular amongst educationalists and which can also be applied to clinical work. If a goal is precisely worded in behavioural terms then it fulfills the criteria normally applied to an objective. Quite simply we do not need both words unless our goals are written in such a way that they fall into an uneasy twilight between aims and objectives.

When planning the treatment of a patient, the first things to establish are the aims. These state the direction and the hoped for result. Without these aims, individual treatment measures can become fragmented and unco-ordinated, a hand-to-mouth process always based on the question 'what shall we do next?'. Having formulated the aims, goals are proposed which will direct and co-ordinate immediate action. These provide a logical basis for planning and a continuous return of information allowing one to keep track of performance against time.

Group activities or events should also have their own aims and goals if they are to merit inclusion within a departmental routine. The aims will reflect the overall purpose of their provision. Their goals will relate to the separate needs of individual patients whose participation has been arranged.

Setting goals

Formulating a treatment goal is not something which is done to a patient in the same way that he may be given an injection or allocated a bed. As far as possible, goals should be set with his comprehension and involvement. How else can he co-operate with their successful achievement? Nor is this a procedure which should be carried out in isolation from other concerned people. If doctors, nurses, family members, ancillary staff, volunteers or anybody else has a part to play then they should at best be involved and at least be informed. The patient is, of course, the most important member of the team responsible for setting goals. Even if he is very disabled it is right for him to know in simple terms what is expected of him and to what end.

A comprehensive goal should contain four separate elements, namely conditions, actions, criteria for success and consequences.

The conditions relate to general events and avoid making assumptions that everything will always go according to plan. They can often be expressed in phrases which start with the words 'providing' or 'given that . . .'. For example:

1. Providing that her husband agrees . . .
2. Given that she has no unexpected visitors . . .
3. Whenever he arrives in the department . . .
4. Providing that the facilities are available . . .

The actions relate to what specified people are going to do. These may include the therapist, the patient or any other individual or group of people. The words used should be precise enough to allow each person to know what they should be doing and, if possible, when this activity should take place. For example:

1. . . . Mrs Smith will cook every meal for the family during the weekend and Mr Smith will not intervene.
2. . . . The student will study for two hours each night.
3. . . . The occupational therapist will greet Fred and initiate conversation with him for five minutes.
4. . . . Emily will show Miss Pigeon how to use the washing machine and they will do the washing together every Monday.

The criterion for success is the measurable part of the goal. It should clearly state what should have been achieved. Care needs to be taken to avoid using abstract concepts which do not allow distinction between success and having to think again. If possible a time limit should be included in order to prevent unsuccessful tactics being continued indefinitely. For example:

1. The family will be served with freshly cooked meals.
2. By Friday she will be able to describe accurately the chemical transmission of nerve impulses over synapses.
3. Fred will begin to greet other people and to make spontaneous comments or enquiries by Christmas.
4. After 6 weeks Miss Pigeon will be able to sort and launder correctly all her own clothes.

Consequences arise from these results and relate to stages in the achievement of aims. If we know what has happened in terms of success or failure then we need to think about what this means in terms of future planning. There are, of course, negative and positive consequences which could be added to every goal. A better perspective is usually gained by looking at short term rather than long term effects.

Examples of negative consequences:
1. If Mrs Smith cannot manage cooking at home over a weekend, her discharge from hospital must be delayed while plans are made for a greater degree of continuing support.

2. If she cannot do this and subsequently fails the physiology test she must seek aid in changing her method and place of study.

Examples of positive consequences:

3. If this improvement in communication occurs Fred will be referred to the training group in social skills.

4. Miss Pigeon will remain within the training programme for a group home and will now start to use the laundrette when she goes shopping each week.

This whole process may sound like a rather complicated game of consequences, which is the nearest parallel which comes to mind. It is, however, an important game, without which staff and patients may waste time in unproductive pursuits or in activities which are carried out without due regard for their effectiveness. It is particularly difficult to set goals relating to social behaviours, such as forming relationships or gaining confidence, but it is not impossible. Inevitably the conditions, actions and consequences suffer in precision from the inclusion of more abstract terms but this need not matter if the criteria for success are made clear and measurable.

The only way to learn to formulate useful goals for patients is to practise and to expose your attempts to colleagues who will discuss, modify and support them. The most common fault is to try to embrace too much within a goal. It is better to isolate skills and to be modest in ambition in order to build on success, rather than to set yourself and your patient an impossibly complex task with rewards that are too distant to contemplate.

It is not sufficient to be aware of goals within one's own thinking and not to set them down or communicate them to others. Such a practice leads to two great temptations, first that of identifying goals retrospectively and second that of failing to examine and adjust programmes of treatment at regular intervals.

Personal goals

Everyone can set their own goals, in either a formal or an informal way, which establish recognizable milestones towards the fulfilment of personal aims or ambitions. It is as important that staff should identify their own professional goals as that they should become proficient in formulating goals for patients. If you do not consider the organisation of your own time and behaviour, its desired results and the criteria you would apply to determine success, then it becomes all too easy just to dribble on from day to day. If you have good reasons for 'just dribbling on' then these should be stated, if only to relieve the pressures of guilt and boredom. When insurmountable barriers present themselves it is helpful to be able to assess how much of the problem presented is related to your own performance and how much to genuinely external influences. Not achieving a specified goal does not necessarily imply failure, it merely signals that reconsideration and the use of a little imagination have become due. At the end of a year you may find that you have 'scored' on seventy per cent of planned possibilities, missed a handful of promising penalties and are attempting to justify injury time through to the following March. But at least you knew what you were trying to achieve and how you intended to set about it.

As a practice exercise try taking one of the following aims and proposing preliminary goals which are within your own capability:

1. To grow cyclamen plants from seed.
2. To give up occupational therapy and become an internationally acclaimed opera singer.

It will be noticed that these two general aims differ in dimension and complexity. One may take longer to achieve, or be more realistic than the other, depending on previous experience and talent. Both can be broken down to goals which include conditions, actions, criteria for success and consequences.

The goals of a practising occupational therapist are more likely to concern knowledge to be gained, arrangements to be made, information to be recorded or sessions of treatment to be carried out. The therapist's clinical goals may be closely related to those of individual patients.

Patients may have in mind their own aims and goals, depending on the degree of motivation and autonomy that they have retained. These may be realistic, or otherwise, depending on the capabilities and insight of the individual. It is the therapist's task to help the patient first of all to express his intentions and then to modify or formulate these in a way which can be understood, accepted and acted upon. It is very difficult, however well intentioned, to impose goals on another person without being able to demonstrate clearly the context. It is the patient's motivation, as much as the therapist's, which is essential to achievement. It may be easier to agree certain suggested aims, such as leaving hospital, going on holiday, gaining privileges, participating in social events or performing a recognized job. In the context of such aims the formulation of more specific goals has some mutual purpose and can become a shared responsibility.

MAKING PROGRESS

If all relevant information has been obtained and organized, if the aims are realistic and the goals correctly formulated, then actually planning a programme is extraordinarily easy.

Returning to the diagram of boxes at the beginning of the chapter we have to consider the use of the environment (Ch. 9), the activity (Ch. 11) and the therapist. Two further considerations within planning are organisation of time and deployment of staff, including qualified therapists, students, helpers and volunteers.

Recapitulation

At the point at which treatment is being planned the therapist should be able to bring together many of the threads which have been discussed so far. These are the questions to which answers should be known.

1. What is the extent of the patient's present disability?
2. Which problems have been identified for intervention by occupational therapy?
3. What particular attitudes or attributes of the patient will influence relationships or activities within treatment?
4. What are the priorities within treatment?
5. Have baselines of performance or behaviour been established?

6. What are the present aims of treatment?
7. Can preliminary but specific goals be stated?
8. Is treatment to be based on learning theory, developmental deficits, social relationships or the gaining of personal insight?
9. What is the amount of time available?
10. What other treatment is he receiving?

The trouble with text books is that they seem to relate only to an ideal world. There are some very real reasons for being unable to answer these questions. These include the 'inheritance' of large numbers of patients whose needs have not received individual attention in the recent past; the acceptance of 'blanket referrals' of all patients irrespective of their suitability for occupational therapy; the lack of staff who can select, assess and make plans for individual patients. If such problems exist then the first priority is to reduce numbers of patients to a reasonable ratio with the number of staff. This may require the provision of diversional activities for those not selected for immediate active treatment. Such a re-arrangement may be essential if any effective treatment is to be carried out.

Organisation of time

There are about 36 hours in most people's working week. Within this total each therapist needs to define sessions for treatment and assessment, time for preparation and for recording, time for communication with other staff (for example during wardrounds, conferences or teaching sessions) and time for personal professional development. Time devoted to the treatment of patients should obviously be the priority. Frustration tends to increase when time devoted to one of the major responsibilities gets out of balance with the others. Proportionate allocation of time will depend on the responsibilities of individual members of staff but it is hard to justify the tendency for greater experience or seniority leading to lesser contact with patients and more administrative duties.

The patient is unlikely to be short of time, his day may begin early and, apart from complying with routine, may really be very dull in hospital.

Within an institution plans should be made to give him opportunity for purposeful activity for at least the equivalent of a working day, even if this is not all spent with occupational therapy. Patients living in the community may require less timetabled activity since they have domestic responsibilities and travel to contend with.

Within each day there are 'normal' times for being engaged in different types of activity. Work and learning are appropriate to the earlier parts of the day and more social or recreational pursuits to late afternoon, evening or weekends.

This may seem a bit conventional but it does echo the practices of the general society to which the patient may hopefully return. If patients are engaged in industrial work during the day it may be more appropriate to develop social skills or domestic ability at other times. If working traditional hours on weekdays does not provide the most rational and effective service for patients then more occupational therapists should be encouraged to alter their routine. Early morning and evening and empty weekends all have their potential for development. Professional concern means knowing what your patient does on a long Sunday afternoon, but it can also mean staying in bed on a Monday morning. Ask the nursing staff, they know what it is all about.

Deployment of staff

Occupational therapy departments may be poor in the number of qualified staff but can be rich in potential resources of alternatively skilled people. These may include helpers, technicians, specialists such as potters, artists and beauticians, nursing students, volunteers and others. Occupational therapy students may have specific objectives of their own for learning but have individual skills to offer as well. Each person needs to be engaged in duties which use his potential fully and which demand the appropriate level of accountability. Occupational therapists should be specifically involved in the treatment of patients. Helpers, technicians and other specialists should be mainly engaged in the provision of activity which can be used by the therapist as a part of treatment. For example, if a potter runs a pottery workshop, a technician a woodwork unit, a helper runs domestic and craft classes and a volunteer organises the vegetable patch, the occupational therapist is free to work in any of these places with selected patients. A wise therapist may even employ a helper to do routine administrative work, control stock and keep interruptions to treatment, such as the telephone, under control.

Student nurses and other temporary staff need to be allowed to develop a specific role in the department. Observation in itself can become dull unless directed by being told what to look for and punctuated by periods of more tangible activity.

A great deal of thought has to be devoted to using each available person in a positive way and inevitably the therapist charged with controlling such activity must steer a path somewhere between departmental anarchy and sitting in the office all day deciding what other people should do.

The programme

Given the range of activities and staff available, a timetable needs to be devised for each patient or group of patients. It may be convenient to divide time spent within occupational therapy into a number of sessions during the morning, afternoon or evening. The length of each session should be determiend by the stamina and span of concentration which is characteristic of the patients concerned. Not all of the patient's time will be spent within occupational therapy; he may be involved in treatment provided by other members of the team or in recreational activities.

A well balanced timetable needs to include sessions of work or learning, social opportunities and time spent in personal or domestic activity. The patient needs to know in advance what he will be doing. If this information is not available to him then his obvious alternatives are passive concurrence or active refusal. Where his personal aims and goals allow a choice of activity this should be offered beforehand.

The occupational therapist who arranges a programme of activity is well placed to understand its complexity or rationale. This does not mean that it is as clear to patients or to other staff. It is often helpful to provide a patient with a written timetable of his proposed activities as an adjunct to discussion. Programmes should also be displayed in wards and in activity areas so that everyone knows who, and what, to expect.

If aims and goals are kept continually under review, there should be no danger of a programme becoming static. Staff can, however, become 'stale' if their own activities are not also reviewed and subject to rotation. This problem is accentuated when the capability of the patients is less than that of the staff concerned. Careful planing, therefore, should provide challenges and new experiences for staff as well as the patients, and provide, for both, a balanced variety within each day.

The weekly programme for each patient should include a specified time set aside for discussion with his therapist about his activities and his progress. For similar reasons each member of staff needs to have time allotted to discussion with a more experienced colleague in order to keep the use of time and abilities under review.

BIBLIOGRAPHY

Kushlick A, Blunden R, Horner D, Smith J 1975 Goal setting in the handicapped person in the community. Course text. The Open University, Milton Keynes
Reed K, Sanderson S 1980 Concepts of occupational therapy. Williams and Wilkins, Baltimore

RECOMMENDED READING

Day D J 1973 A systems diagram for teaching treatment planning. American Journal of Occupational Therapy 27: 5, 239–243
Hume C, Pullen I 1986 Rehabilitation in psychiatry. Churchill Livingstone, Edinburgh
Line J 1969 Case method as a scientific form of clinical thinking. American Journal of Occupational Therapy 27: 5, 239–243

9

The environment

One of the first and most significant therapeutic tools is the environment provided or influenced by the therapist. This does not mean purely the physical resources and style of a department or unit but includes the prevalent attitudes or ethos within the patient's surroundings. Thousands of pounds' worth of light airy space filled with bright ideas, videotape equipment, flourishing pot plants and cheerful encouragement may be no more therapeutic than the inconvenient little huts where many occupational therapy departments started. Nor will any amount of frenetic activity guarantee that the environment is one in which patients feel that they have the opportunity and ability to act. This does not mean that space and equipment are unimportant. It does mean that one cannot really know what is needed in physical terms without an understanding of what one is trying to provide or to achieve in more abstract terms. It is true that someone has to devote time to managerial politics, planning and stock control, but the clinical therapists addressed here should regard their more important role as being part of a therapeutic environment. Good administration involves not being in the office during sessions of treatment.

The environment must first of all be different from the regimes experienced by the patient elsewhere. It is a normal

146

expectation to be exposed to different situations in the course of each day. Moving between different environments allows an individual to vary and to extend his behaviour; he has opportunities to relate to people in different ways, to exercise a range of abilities and to take on different roles. Look back to Chapter 3 on the 'development of self' and the way in which the identity of an individual can stem from his involvement within a variety of environmental and social contexts. The role of occupational therapy within a large institution includes attempting to provide such a variety.

One of the intentions often stated by therapists is that of 'providing stimulation'. This chapter will, first of all, consider some of the implications of stimulation and learning within occupational therapy and then look at some of the environments which may be involved.

STIMULATION

A stimulus in this context is something that rouses someone to activity, that excites him. The resultant activity may be physical or mental. One can be stimulated through all the sensory channels, visual, auditory, tactile, olfactory, gustatory and kinesthetic, separately or together. A teacher may try to integrate two channels to stimulate learning by providing visual material in conjunction with the spoken word. A therapist may try to stimulate activity by providing a range of examples, a choice of materials or a setting in which much other activity is going on. Before getting too enthusiastic about providing maximum stimulation for all patients one should consider exactly what this entails and whether it is always appropriate. If it means being subjected to an artificially high quantity of sensory information, randomly presented, this may even be counter productive. It presupposes three abilities:

1. To attend selectively to stimuli
2. To habituate to constant stimuli so that they become 'background'
3. To integrate information from different sensory channels.

Most people are able to attend to stimulation in this way

but we have already mentioned in Chapter 6 the schizophrenic patient who may not. He appears to have problems
in receiving sensory information at a level at which he can
deal with it and experiences problems related to a high level
of cortical arousal.

Groups of patients for whom one might argue the need for
maximum stimulation are those who have some form of
cerebral damage, for example, the mentally handicapped, and
some of the elderly severely mentally ill. The severely
mentally handicapped, like small children, are easily
distracted, having very short spans of concentration. An
environment in which a variety of stimuli are continually available — sound, colour, movement and touch — may enrich
their experience and facilitate development towards their
potential.

Programmes to orient patients towards reality have been
instigated for elderly patients suffering from cerebral deterioration. These consist of a highly stimulating physical
environment coupled with regular presentation of information about time, place, personal details and immediate
events.

The argument against regarding maximum stimulation
simplistically as a method of treatment for these groups of
patients is that success is less likely to rely on the quantity of
stimulation than upon its selection and presentation. Bear in
mind the effects of familiarity, also remembering as an
example that the continuous playing of popular music can
give rise to as much irritation and apathy as benefit. The
suggestion therefore is that we drop this concept of
'maximum stimulation' as being generally useful and discuss
'selective stimulation' as an alternative.

Selective stimulation

There are two obvious ways of eliminating extraneous input
in order to allow an individual to attend selectively. One is
to limit stimuli to one sensory modality at one time, for
example talking or playing music in the absence of visual
distractions or any other simultaneous activity. The other is
to limit subject matter, for example if a patient is being taught
to use a printing press, or perform any other task, visual,

auditory and tactile senses may be involved together but other irrelevant information emanating from people, decorations and activities can be physically excluded.

The programme of 'reality orientation' will involve each of the five senses; activities can be devised to re-introduce and identify familiar smells, tastes and textures whilst eliminating visual or auditory cues. If the group of patients are involved in discussion then this should be arranged so as not to have competition from other noises or activities. A clock, a calender or the label on a door should not be masked by the proximity of other notices or decorations. If the radio or television is used it needs to be switched on and off, the content of the programme being reinforced or expanded in other ways, rather than being continually present as a background feature of the environment.

Areas which are specific to a limited range of activities such as kitchens, art rooms, quiet rooms and other rooms designed for personal care, workshop activities, clerical skills or recreation have obvious advantages. Each can be made relevant to its purpose, stimulating participation rather than confusion. Where large multipurpose rooms are employed there is a temptation to fill them with a cheerful array of materials, equipment, completed projects and posters. It is difficult to create a balance. On the one hand it is important to provide a characteristic atmosphere which is different from a ward or clinic and which suggests opportunity and activity. On the other hand an aura of confusion or the general appearance of a primary school holding a jumble sale may not be helpful to a patient who is sensitive of his adult status or is easily distracted. A compromise may be to create an information area and to design good clear displays which can be used and removed. Partitions may be helpful to subdivide a large space or to enclose areas which can then develop their own characteristic appearance and atmosphere.

Working with depressed patients a prime object may be to stimulate them in any way, to rouse the individual from subjective feelings of hopelessness, inability or unhappiness. The idea of limiting stimulation to a level where it can be selected and presented relevantly remains useful even if the choice of activity is relatively unimportant. These patients often have difficulty in making decisions and plans and judging merit. By controlling the environment it becomes possible to grade a function such as making decisions from a simple dichotomy such as stating a preference between green and blue to the complex planning of personal activities.

Optimum levels of stimulation in schizophrenia

The possible influence of different levels of social stimulation on the symptoms of schizophrenia were discussed in Chapter 6. In simple terms an impoverished environment tends to increase the symptoms of the defects such as emotional flatness, withdrawal and difficulty in formulating plans and decisions. The patient in this sort of environment appears to be less capable and more institutionalized. An emotionally demanding and stimulating environment, such as may be present in an over energetic programme of rehabilitation or a highly charged home environment following discharge, may increase the florid symptoms such as delusions, confused thought and disturbed behaviour. The schizophrenic patient requires an optimal environment in order to function as well as possible, that is one in which both these extremes are avoided.

This obviously has relevance to an occupational therapist engaged in devising a programme of treatment and designing an environment in which these programmes may be carried out successfully.

Too little social stimulation is likely to be a greater problem than too much, whilst the patient is living within an institution. It is very hard to motivate a patient towards activity when the typical schizophrenic syndrome tends to result in inertia. Additionally, the environment may appear to the schizophrenic patient to be particularly chaotic or incomprehensible since he may be attending indiscriminately to relevant and irrelevant stimuli. This suggests that the most successful attempts at stimulation must be clear, unambiguous and made directly to the individual patient. The intrinsic anarchy of the schizophrenic world may indicate why behavioural methods can be useful in stimulating activity. A simple proposition of cause and effect is made. 'You will participate in this specified activity and as a direct result you will receive this specified reward'.

The therapist should present a wide variety of selected stimuli in an attempt to overcome inertia and social withdrawal. Individual sessions between the patient and the therapist are useful in that communication can be specific, direct and undistracted; however these should be kept fairly low-key so that the patient is stimulated but not confronted or pressurized. Activities in small groups enable the patient to act in co-operation with others and to involve himself as much as he is able to without being the continual focus of attention. It is more difficult genuinely to stimulate the individual patient in the context of a large group for more than a fraction of the time unless a high ratio of skilled and observant staff are included in the group.

As rehabilitation progresses, and as discharge to a normal world is contemplated, the patient must learn to recognize and respond to social causes and effects of far greater complexity. The degree and type of stimulation to which he has been subjected has been monitored by the therapist. This has been designed to gain his participation whilst avoiding exposing him to a degree of personal intrusion which he can not cope with. In order to continue to benefit from such an optimum environment the patient must learn to monitor his own involvement. For patients in later stages of rehabilitation, therefore, the therapist needs deliberately to reduce the protective aspects of controlling or selecting stimulation.

Relinquishing control

Still in the context of the schizophrenic, there are a number of things this patient needs to learn in addition to the familiar range of practical skills. He must learn to anticipate and avoid situations which could have unhealthy results for him. He must be able to select companions who will understand his condition sufficiently not to intrude upon him. He must learn to withdraw in a controlled way from situations which are socially dangerous to him so that he can return to participation at will. If he can start to develop these skills within the hospital, including the occupational therapy department, he must also recognize what he is learning so that he can apply this understanding to other situations.

The way in which this can be achieved depends on the

individual patient and the staff and on the opportunities presented, but the patient may be considered individually or within a small group. In the first instance the patient may be involved in planning his own activities for each day and discussing with the therapist the reason for his choices, his response to situations as they have arisen and any deductions that he has been able to make from the experience. Such discussions should be kept factual and supportive and directed towards simple illumination rather than intensity of emotional response. Other patients may find small discussion groups with similarly disabled patients more appropriate. Recognition of mutual difficulties and suggestions as to how they can be overcome may form part of the final programme for patients just before discharge or be included in the later sessions of a group receiving training in social skills.

It is not only the schizophrenic patient who needs to regain control over his own environment. Personal freedom in choice of activity and mode of social interaction should only be reduced during a period when a patient is unable to act positively in his own interests. For example, the depressed patient may find it difficult to exercise personal choice or to motivate himself towards either any activity or general health whilst he is predominantly miserable. Unaided he may attempt tasks or expose himself to situations which will reinforce his sense of failure and worthlessness; alternatively he may maintain his existing patterns of distress and inaccessability. However, if his environment continues to be controlled or over-manipulated after he has recovered sufficiently to practise a degree of autonomy, how can he ever regain self respect and the ability to manage his own life with confidence?

One could continue to use examples from a wide range of patient's problems to illustrate the need to monitor the environment and the degree of control which contributes to that environment. There are, though, two main points which need to be emphasized. If it is necessary to intervene, through control or selection of experience, in someone else's life, then it is necessary to relinquish that control as part of the same therapy. There can be valid therapeutic reasons for controlling a patient's environment. However, when patients stay in hospital for a long time or tend to be dependent, the basis of these controls can slip from what is beneficial to the patient to what is expedient for the staff. Every decision made by staff, whether related to the activities of one patient or the routine of many, needs to be constantly reviewed in this light.

TEACHING AND LEARNING

The therapist is an intrinsic part of the therapeutic environment. Teaching is part of the therapist's role, a part that not only includes but also exceeds involvement in behaviour modification and the technical teaching of skills. Patients attend an occupational therapy department in order to learn, but again, this should be given a wide interpretation. One does not only learn specific functions or pieces of behaviour; given the opportunity one can also acquire knowledge about oneself and about how to survive in a wider society. All therapists should be aware of strategies to maximize an environment for learning and this involves knowledge of some education theory. In addition to providing a learning environment for patients, most therapists are involved in the teaching of students from their own and from other disciplines, so an awareness of how effective learning takes place becomes doubly relevant.

Active learning

Being the passive recipient of information is not as effective a method of learning as being actively involved. Consider which group of student nurses will understand most about occupational therapy; the group which receives a lecture on the subject or the group which is involved within a dynamic and well-run department? Or, if a group is exposed to a superb lecture and a boring or muddled practical experience, which of these will be the greater influence on their memory as recalled 6 months later?

Information can be given about simple laws, such as that, in a right-angled triangle, the square of the hypotenuse is equal to the sum of the squares of the other two sides, or that vacuum cleaners cease to suck efficiently if the bag is not emptied. Such information becomes meaningful when the

learner puts it into practice and experiences its consequences. There is limited value in delivering 'talks' to patients
on subjects such as domestic economy, self-care, social
behaviour or employment. Well considered doses of initial
guidance or factual information need to be followed by
activity which applies the skills or information involved.

Practice is essential to acquiring skills or to memorizing
information, but such practice is most valuable when reinforcement, or advice regarding the improvement of performance, is also available. Repetition without such responses is
less effective when learning new behaviours. The less able the
learner the more care should be taken in spacing out
rehearsal and recall. In a programme which involves the
acquisition of a large range of skills, each skill must have
'rehearsal time' built into subsequent parts of the programme.
To fabricate a simple example, in a programme lasting 12
calendar months in which use of public telephones was
covered in March, this skill needs to be regularly utilized
between April and December. The therapist cannot cross it
off as 'done' even though the learners could perform the task
adequately after initial teaching. Each time this skill, or any
other, is performed the learner should receive back information about its effectiveness or about any improvements
which could still be made.

When the material to be learnt is more abstract, such as
being able to open one's mind to another's point of view, the
same principles apply. It is no good telling someone that they
ought to be more receptive. Situations or discussions need
to be created through which the ability can be developed
gradually, and back through which the learner's increasing
ability can be reflected.

People learn through each other and not just through the
formal vehicle of a teacher or a therapist. This is fortunate
since, were it not so, we should be expected to know all the
answers. A therapist can be at a disadvantage, being not
disabled, not confronted by social inadequacies and fears, not
dependent on the goodwill of others and not fearful of the
future. People who are socially or emotionally handicapped
have experiences and knowledge that we cannot always
share. Remember Erving Goffman in Chapter 3 — we may be
the 'wise' but we are not the 'own'. This is one of the factors

upon which we base treatment in groups. Each member can share problems, experience, and tentative solutions from first-hand knowledge. Such material can be tested by patients through direct application to their own situation.

Principles not answers

Practical living involves a wide range of skills but one cannot hope to provide a predetermined solution for every problem that a patient may meet. This is why a programme of re-habilitation based purely on the teaching of skills cannot be genuinely comprehensive. Individuals survive in society by being able to function within a variety of roles and by being able to solve problems. They also survive by recognizing those problems which they are likely to be unable to solve, and by seeking the appropriate help. Some people can resolve their own marital difficulties but cannot unblock drains or fill in income tax forms, others may have a different pattern of competence in solving problems. Essentially one needs some confidence in one's own personal skills, some realization of one's deficits and some knowledge of where to turn to for help.

The principles which an individual uses to solve practical and personal problems may be embedded partly in science or technology, partly in a personal doctrine or system of beliefs, and partly in experience. These three factors may make uneasy bedfellows but each in a way impinges on the nature and provision of therapy.

The first is the most straightforward; it is a part of teaching practical skills to impart the principles underlying personal and domestic hygiene, efficient working and personal organ-isation. Few moral dilemmas arise from protecting the body from disease or decay, the living area from uncomfortable chaos or personal administration from disorganization. These skills can be taught and can be related to empirical knowledge.

Therapists may be a little more tentative about beliefs or about morality as useful guiding concepts, although they apply these to making decisions within their own lives. This could be either because such concepts are unfashionable or because they are less easy to define. Certainly personal convictions are difficult to mesh with therapy, perhaps because in common with other medical colleagues we make a priority of finding scientifically respectable solutions to problems which can include spiritual distress. This is a tricky area, but a therapist can start by examining the basis of his or her own code of conduct.

Being able to identify one's own personal beliefs or morality can gain one the freedom not to impose these upon others but to recognise a fellow individual's need to have his own personal philosophy or security. This can involve putting aside one's own degree of faith, agnosticism or confusion and being alert to the needs and the capabilities of the disabled person being served. Thus there are occasions when churches, associations, adoptive relatives and other individuals who are not medically oriented may be able to offer something that the professionals cannot. When we do identify needs which we cannot fulfill, it can require both wisdom and courage to seek help for the patient from some more appropriate person.

Most therapists have the third factor — experience. We deal with unexpected and unsolicited events almost every day. There is a power cut or a bus strike, a door to door salesman is over-persistent, the neighbours complain, a circular promises beauty and intelligence for £19.95, someone refuses a reasonable request, the gas bill arrives, and you cope. What about the patient who has a history of not being able to cope and who is once more to be discharged to independent or to partially sheltered living? The answer to each hypothetical situation cannot be given within a programme of rehabilitation. One is dealing with individuals who, whatever their diagnosis, are unusually vulnerable within society. Giving people experience as a practical exercise inevitably involves a degree of simulation and therefore of unreality. Contrived experience can, however, be useful in starting to develop skills in solving problems. The simplest type of exercise can involve discovering factual information; for example obtaining specified facts from other patients, from staff or from newspapers. Patients may use facilities in the community to find out about comparative prices in shops, forthcoming events, times and costs of entertainments or how to reach a number of stated destinations.

Discussions within groups and 'role play' can be used to examine a range of responses to different social or practical situations. These can vary from coping with inquisitive acquaintances, or answering personal questions from employers or authorities, to acquiring help from the various agencies available in the community.

During later stages of treatment patients may be placed in more comprehensive simulated environments such as self-contained flats within the hospital. Within such units they should be able to discover how to establish their own daily routines, organize their own catering and entertainment, budget adequately and generally take care of themselves and their immediate environment at a level which they find comfortable. Although this type of arrangement sounds ideal, some units with these general objectives fail to provide a realistic degree of separation from the regime of the institution. Staff who are there, in theory only in case of difficulty, tend to make themselves over-available to the patients. A piece of friendly advice which is offered only as a suggestion is likely to be interpreted as an instruction, if only because it comes from someone who previously has controlled the patient and his environment. It is also difficult not to impose one's own standards of order and hygiene on patients in such a semi-independent situation. They may enjoy the freedom of living in a bit of a muddle and letting the washing-up accumulate — a lot of apparently normal people do. The therapist, as a teacher, must learn to discriminate between a patient who can apply principles to solving the problems of living in his own way and one who is unready to cope with the organisational and emotional aspects of independence.

SPECIFIC ENVIRONMENTS

Every environment develops in a different way according to the eccentric needs of its users. There are a number of different types of unit which may be involved in the treatment of long stay psychiatric patients. The following descriptions of some of these are brief and merely indicate the range of facilities which should be investigated when considering the scope of a programme of rehabilitation. They should also illustrate the close relationship between rehabilitative measures and the environment in which they are carried out. In some cases it can be argued that the provision of a particular environment is the major form of treatment and not just a setting for activity.

Industrial units

Industrial work may be undertaken by patients as a progressive form of treatment or in order to maintain a maximum level of ability and health. Within hospitals, industrial units may be run by occupational therapists, by nurses or by other suitably qualified or experienced staff. In the community there may be industrial therapy organisations, firms or organisations offering sheltered work, day centres using work activities, employment rehabilitation centres, skills centres or other facilities for training and education. The provisions vary from area to area so it is important to investigate locally the contributions of the local authority, the health service, education, voluntary organisations and industry.

The value of work in rehabilitation lies in the concept that work is a normal activity which can at its best be associated with status, reward, satisfaction and acceptability. This implies that the work available to a patient should be selected and presented in order to maximise these associations. The organisation of work activities will be considered in the next chapter but the source of work and the conditions under which it is performed are both relevant here. To be most effective work should be realistic and be of some recognisable value to society. An apparently pointless task, one which is unnecessary or has no recognizable product, is unlikely to contribute toward an environment which promotes self-respect and constructive behaviour.

Work may be obtained on contract from outside industry and include tasks such as light assembly, packaging or retrieving parts. It may be generated by the needs of a hospital such as work from the central stores sterilizing department, the printing of forms or cards; or work, now diminishing in availability, in service departments such as laundry, stores or gardens. Lastly, work may consist of projects created within an industrial unit, such as making garden furniture, manufacturing toys or equipment on a production line, casting concrete slabs or a variety of other propositions.

It is often stated that work or the working environment should be realistic, but what does this really mean? In normal settings both are subject to wide variations and yet remain real enough. There is however little more unrealistic and dismal than an ill-matched group of patients being paid a few pence each week for carelessly performing repetitive tasks in a haze of tobacco smoke and misunderstanding.

If one is simulating a productive workshop then there are some fairly obvious criteria. Standard workshop safety rules should apply, the quality of finished work should be monitored and maintained, stock keeping of materials and products should be systematic and working areas should be adequately equipped and specific to the task. Expectations of the individual related to attendance and responsibilities should be clear and remuneration should reflect performance. Many industrial units are successful in providing this type of basic organisation and at least some attention is paid to grading work, according to its complexity or to the degree of discretion involved, so that patients are given both a variety of work and an opportunity to perform at their highest possible level of ability.

It is difficult to discuss a working environment without mentioning financial rewards. Payment is one of the strongest motivators, not just for industrialists, shopfloor workers and advertisers but for therapists, their medical colleagues and their patients. Even if you can fool yourself that your own motives are purely altruistic and non-material, such a doctrine cannot realistically be imposed on others. Ideally, if work is to provide status and personal satisfaction and a genuine link with a normal lifestyle, wages should have some correlation with money earned in outside industry. There are three main problems which often preclude this:

1. The comparatively low income earned by industrial units because of the type of work which they undertake or the speed at which it can be completed.
2. There is a restriction on the amount a patient may earn before such payments affect any sickness benefit which is receiving.

3. A realistic wage earned within an institution could arguably be balanced against the cost of a patient's board and lodgings and the cost of other services being supplied to him. The ensuing mathematical, ethical and administrative problems could be alarming.

On the other hand it must be realized that, for many patients, inadequate rewards will amount to reduced motivation. Society places a monetary value on people and to deal in pence rather than in pounds can place, in the patient's eyes, a low valuation on his own ability or existence.

The patient may be involved in assessing his own earnings in collaboration with staff using established criteria. Such criteria may include punctuality, attendance, output, responsibility or initiative, personal presentation, level of co-operation with others or any other factors considered relevant to the individual patient or to the unit. The advantages of such a system are that patients are aware of the reasons for variations in their earnings, that they are aware of and involved in setting their own work objectives and that differences in an individual patient's performance as perceived by himself and by staff become a subject for immediate discussion.

Units for the elderly

The adjectives 'geriatric' and psychogeriatric' are diminishing in popularity for the purpose of general description of elderly people. After all, most therapists hope to produce a child rather than a 'paediatric' person at the end of pregnancy and themselves look forward to being 'old' or 'elderly' rather than 'geriatric'. Units for the elderly mentally ill are beginning to reflect this desire to afford dignity and acceptance to aging. A custodial attitude directed by the twin concerns of safety and hygiene used to create barren wards and day-rooms with patients safety seated on the periphery and discouraged from independent movement. Private activities such as bathing, using the toilet and sleeping were made public as a matter of expediency. Confusion was greeted with cheerful tolerance and a conviction that this was inevitable and not causing the sufferer any untoward distress. Recent developments in the care of the elderly have, however, eschewed the route of expediency, safety and hygiene. Instead they have referred back to values traditionally held by the extended family, providing social support, comfort and sensitivity to individual needs.

The environment for caring for the elderly relies upon co-operation and communication between disciplines. The problems of an individual tend to be multiple, including, for example, physical, social and psychiatric problems in addition to the general degenerative effects of aging. Families, doctors, nurses, social workers, occupational therapists and other specialists may all be involved in the management of each person. In general terms the environment of an old person in residential or hospital care needs to include as much privacy as possible, individuality in clothing and personal possessions and a background of normal activity. Forget the well-designed day-rooms overlooking quiet gardens with piped music more suited to a crematorium. Introduce a few unhygienic cats or a parrot and a view of a busy thoroughfare; abandon the starched hats, white coats and brisk coping behaviours. When I'm old and daft and a bit smelly I don't want to be managed tolerantly or to die conveniently. I want to know that my integrity is recognised, feel accepted and at home.

There are practical problems in creating a comfortable environment for elderly mentally infirm patients. Cognitive changes and visuo-spatial difficulties make it hard for an elderly person to find his way around an unfamiliar building, and often confusion may increase as a result of being admitted to hospital. The various measures taken to overcome these problems include colour coding of rooms or lines tiled into floors leading to vital facilities such as the toilet. Such measures are the delight of planners and administrators but they are no substitute for attempting to reduce the degree of confusion experienced by the individual patient.

A method of treatment based on specific use of the environment is known as 'reality orientation'. Those who enjoy being grammatically correct call it 'orientation towards reality'.

Orientation towards reality can be either a policy or a technique. As a policy it means that every interaction with the patient should be used as an opportunity to reinforce concepts such as personal names, time, place and conditions. The patient is always called by name and not by anonymous appellations such as 'dear' or 'love'. The time of day and what is happening are reinforced by constant mention, and details about the unit are constantly repeated. Staff try to be consistent in their approach, a limited number of individuals being made personally known to each patient.

Orientation towards reality as a technique can involve a series of carefully planned sessions with a small group of patients selected for their common degree of confusion. Each session is used to examine and reinforce a familiar concept such as common smells, the current season, food, past personal events or mutual interests — anything, in fact, which is familiar and can be brought to attention from the past rather than presented as entirely new material. The intention is to reinstate existing memories or neural pathways rather than to create new ones. Through such methods the patients' ability to communicate and to cope with the present may be improved and they may gain confidence in their ability to grasp and deal with reality.

The opportunity to reminisce is also important to elderly people since this can demonstrate to them not only their own powers of memory but also past abilities to cope and to change. Self-esteem can be gained on the basis of previous successes or experience. The interest shown by others in their reminiscenses enhance this.

RECOMMENDED READING

Bailey R D 1985 Coping with stress in caring. Blackwell, Oxford
Bennett D 1978 Community psychiatry. British Journal of Psychiatry 132: 209–220
Berger P. Luckman T 1967 The social construction of reality. Penguin Books, Middlesex
Clark D H 1981 Social therapy in psychiatry, 2nd edn. Churchill Livingstone, Edinburgh
Foucault M 1976 Mental illness and psychology. Harper Colophon Books, New York
Lamb H R et al 1976 Community survival for long-term patients. Jossey-Bass, San Francisco
Meacher M 1979 (ed) New methods of mental health care. Pergamon Press, Oxford
Wing J K, Morris B 1981 Handbook of psychiatric rehabilitation practice. Oxford University Press, Oxford

Woods R T, Britton P G 1977 Psychological approaches to the treatment of the elderly. Age and Aging Volume 6: 104–112

Wynne A R 1978 Movable group therapy for institutionalized patients. Hospital and Community Psychiatry 29: 8, 516–519

Yerxa E J 1980 Occupational therapy's role in creating a future climate of caring. American Journal of Occupational Therapy 34: 8, 529–534

10

Activities

THE USE OF ACTIVITIES

The work of the occupational therapist, described so far, has been based mainly on theories, personal perceptions and techniques. Processes such as interviewing, assessing, planning goals, controlling environments and devising programmes can all be regarded as techniques or as personal skills on the part of the therapist. The term 'activity' as used in this chapter refers to things that the patient does, even though his performance may be initiated or guided by the therapist.

Activities are the major therapeutic measures used within occupational therapy. Each activity needs to be selected for its relevance to the functional or personal needs of the patient. The most usually desired results of activity are as follows:

1. Information is gained by the patient through his own participation. This information includes knowledge of his own degree of ability or inability in relation to tools and materials. If the activity involves other people he will receive information about how they perceive him and about the extent to which he can gain pleasure or support from co-operative activity. He can test his own beliefs about himself in relation

to his practical skills, his influence over other people and events and his perception of reality.

2. Information is gained by the therapist through observation of the patient's participation. This information includes the patient's ability to organize himself, to relate to other people and the environment, to use equipment, to persist in a task and to resolve problems.

3. New skills can be learnt or existing skills can be rehearsed or improved. This point relates to the performance of tasks required for personal care, domestic independence, using tools and organizing time.

4. Self-concept can be defined or developed. Activities can be used to extend the roles available to a patient and to give him confidence in his ability to organize, control and complete projects.

5. Physical needs can be fulfilled. Exercise, movement and the practice of gross and fine motor control can assist a patient to gain mastery over his own body and improve his own physical and mental state.

6. Activity can provide a channel for communication and the expression of emotion. Although the creative media are the most obvious examples, any activity which involves co-operation with others also involves opportunities to be influential, to contribute ideas and to be recognized as an individual.

7. Specific cognitive deficits can be improved. Such deficits may be, for example, in concentration, memory, reasoning or orientation.

Analysis of activity

If activities are to be applied specifically, the occupational therapist must be able to examine them critically and identify their component parts and the demands of each part. An activity which is included in a programme of assessment needs to be literally torn to pieces by the therapist first in order that the abilities or qualities demanded within its performance are thoroughly appreciated. If this understanding is not gained by the therapist then the patient's success or failure within the activity will have no precise meaning.

Many programmes of treatment are devised which involve progression of a patient from one activity to another in order to extend his skills. Such programmes rely, for their validity, on the therapist being able to analyse the performance of each activity in terms of complexity and social or emotional demands. To use a simple example, in weightlifting the poundage of each weight is known and when one challenge has been met a further known quantity is added to test and develop strength. In more complex or abstract areas of human ability the demands are less easy to quantify but an exhaustive effort must be made to separate and evaluate each element in order to grade activities.

The analysis of an activity can be considered in two stages, breaking it down into its component parts and evaluating each part.

Breaking down activities

This is relatively straight-forward and is an essential part of teaching. The following information must be identified.

1. The materials needed
2. The tools required
3. The finished result, if any
4. The time required for the whole task
5. The environment which is most suitable
6. Whether it is an activity for an individual or a group
7. The stages in order of completion.

The last point should contain the majority of the detailed information and should separate each of the processes involved. For example, the stages in making a cup of tea, using an electric kettle and tea bags for simplicity, are as follows.

1. Fill the kettle
2. Connect it to a supply of electricity
3. Assemble the crockery, milk and sugar
4. Warm the pot
5. Place the necessary teabags in the pot
6. Pour boiling water into the pot

7. Allow it to brew or mash (depending on your place of origin).

When such a breakdown is used for teaching purposes, each stage should be expanded by stating any key points. For example, the key points in relation to filling the kettle would include disconnecting the power, using fresh water, covering the element and replacing the lid with the steam vent directed away from the handle.

Analysing each part

The format for the analysis of activity will depend on the theoretical frame of reference being applied. Behaviour modification requires an emphasis on identifying measurable elements in the performance which can subsequently be re-inforced. An activity to be included in a programme based on personal development will be examined for its potential for self-expression and relationships with others.

The following list gives examples of the range of features which should be relevant to a therapist who is selecting activities for use with long-term patients.

1. Physical demands
   a. Fine motor control — including co-ordination between hand and eye and precise control of tools
   b. Gross motor control — including walking, running, co-ordinating all parts of the body and maintaining balance
   c. Endurance — to standing, to extended periods of activity and of discomfort
   d. Type of movement — unilateral, bilateral, involving bending, stretching, rhythm or speed
   e. Strength
2. Cognitive demands
   a. Concentration
   b. Memory
   c. Use of reasoning to solve problems
   d. Numeracy and literacy
   e. Orientation
   f. Organisation
   g. Use of abstract thought or imagination

3. Sensory and perceptional qualities
   a. Visual — including comprehension of figure-ground, spatial awareness, appreciation of colour, tone and form
   b. Auditory — including selective attention, use of auditory cues, comprehension of language
   c. Kinesthetic — including touch, differentiation of textures, sensations of movement and of awareness of body
   d. Olfactory
   e. Gustatory
4. Social demands
   a. Individual or co-operative activity
   b. Necessity to be aware of others
   c. Sharing tools and ideas
   d. Dependence on verbal communication
   e. Responsibility for others
5. Expressive opportunities
   a. Destructiveness and hostility
   b. Inventiveness and originality
   c. Reflection of present mood
   d. Expression of attitudes and perceptions
   e. Exploring the meaning of feelings
6. Independence
   a. Ability to plan and organize
   b. Involvement of initiative
   c. Degree of dependence on therapist or others
   d. Decisions
   e. Personal application
7. Practical considerations
   a. Tools and materials
   b. Environmental requirements
   c. Noise and dirt
8. Potential for grading
   a. Can be simplified
   b. Can be altered to emphasize specific demand
   c. Can progress in complexity.

Each activity mentioned in the remainder of this chapter can be analysed by the occupational therapist who is considering its potential application. Useful and more comprehensive descriptions of the analysis of activities can be found within Hopkins & Smith (1978) and Llorens (1976) as well as within journals of occupational therapy.

PHYSICAL ACTIVITIES

Exercise

Within Chapter 6 the posture and restrictions in mobility of the schizophrenic patient were mentioned. Many exercises can be devised which directly affect these problems and which may give the patient specific stimulation as well as improving his general health. In the early stages of treatment a low ratio of patients to members of staff can help to encourage full participation. Only when motivation towards this type of activity has been established can the patient afford to join the back row of an existing exercise session. Physical exercises for schizophrenic patients should include those which encourage movements of the head and neck, movements of the limbs across the midline, reaching and stretching. All these activities are atypical of many patients' habitual position and range. Activities which encourage these movements include passing objects over the head or between the legs, ball games, mirroring another person's movements, skipping, pulling on ropes and floor work with discarded parachutes.

The elderly may have physical problems or general frailty to contend with but should still be involved in physical activities in order to maintain strength, mobility, circulation and general health. Suitable activities may be more gentle and include exercises carried out from a sitting position. It is important to involve all parts of the body, and music may be a useful source of stimulation. In addition to formalized exercise sessions, physical movement should be encouraged as much as possible, for instance by visiting a shop or serving each other at meal times, so that the elderly patient needs to get up from a chair at regular intervals.

Mentally handicapped people may have excess physical energy to use up through sport or exercises, but equal attention should be paid to problems of co-ordination. Emphasis should be given to the differences between fast and slow movements, between tension and relaxation and between curling up and stretching out. An awareness of what the body is doing and how it can be controlled precedes the ability to use it in a co-ordinated and expressive way.

Whichever group of patients is being treated, there are certain precautions to take when using physical exercise. Discomfort and distress can arise through exercising in heavy or constricting clothing and muscular strains can be the result of energetic activity which has not been preceded by proper preparation and warming up. A therapist should always be aware of an individual's physical problems or vulnerabilities before engaging him in strenous activity.

Relaxation

Relaxation is not so much the opposite of activity as its complementary state. The real opponent of relaxation is unproductive tension, that feeling of unease and muscular preparedness which is tiring without being effective. Many patients suffer from unproductive tension and need to learn to alter their own physical state in order to free energy for more useful activity. Standard methods of training in relaxation involve alternately tensing and releasing different groups of muscles in turn, in order to gain an awareness of the difference between a tense and a relaxed state. Once a patient is able to discriminate between these states he is better able to use conscious controls over his own body. Such training is sometimes augmented by the use of bio-feedback equipment which gives the patient immediate information about his own degree of muscular tension. Many therapists suggest to patients soothing mental images, or use music to encourage a sense of calm.

Some patients are unable to take full advantage of such training due to a limitation in their span of concentration, an inability to think in abstract terms or to difficulties in applying methods of relaxation to episodes of stress within their own lives. A further problem can be demonstrated by patients who are able to co-operate sufficiently to go to sleep during relaxation sessions but who therefore fail to learn to apply such methods autonomously.

Learning to relax, in a physical sense, is an important part of learning to control anxiety. Long-term patients suffer as much as anyone else from anxiety but may be unable to express this as well as to control it.

For these patients, initial training sessions in relaxation should be brief and should follow periods of more strenous activity in order to provide a more dramatic contrast. Plenty of time should be allowed for discussion to make the concepts of tension and relaxation fully understood. Patients should be encouraged to identify their personal signs of tension, such as raised shoulders, heads that are poked forwards, tightly flexed arms or clenched fists. It is much better to hold a brief daily session which can build up into a full routine of relaxation than to regard this as a weekly event.

SOCIAL ACTIVITIES

The ability to communicate effectively with others is central to all forms of social activity. Someone who is psychiatrically disabled usually has related disorders or limitations in his social contact with others. When any of us are temporarily depressed, anxious or low in self-esteem our relationships with others are affected, often by tendencies to become withdrawn, over-demanding or unreceptive. A person who has long-standing psychiatric problems is likely to have a severely impaired social life. In many cases, odd behaviour or a gradual withdrawal from contact with families and friends may result in a social isolation which precedes any attempt at treatment. Elderly people who are living alone may develop problems as a result of the lack of social contact.

Social activities form a major part of occupational therapy. In addition to providing specific training in social skills, therapists draw widely on the arts as media for treatment. Recreational activities which encourage communication and collaboration also form an important part of the programme. Of course there are very few activities which do not have some social content; those described here have been selected because their primary purpose is to improve or encourage communication.

The arts

Creative activities, such as drawing, painting, modelling, writing and music are all forms of expression. They can not always replace the spoken word but they can stimulate and structure ideas. The ability to explain one's perceptions and anxieties with satisfactory clarity entails a sophisticated use of language and degree of conceptional thinking. Many patients do not have these assets and need time, a secure setting, and an alternative medium in which to express their feelings.

The occupational therapist working with long-term patients need not be concerned with the debatable diagnostic value of art, this is, whether the artistic expression of a patient can be directly correlated with his diagnosis of schizophrenia, organic impairment, depression or personality disorder. Many therapists would claim to recognize a style of painting, for example, as being typical of the work of patients who share a specific range of psychiatric problems. This is hardly surprising since the arts, throughout history, have developed for the purpose of conveying moods, emotions or ways of thinking. When the arts are used within therapy, the emphasis is on the value of the activity and the communication which it stimulates at the time and not on the later analysis of the finished result.

Drawing, painting and collage

A crude but useful distinction can be made between art which is intended to be hung on the wall and art which is destined for the waste paper bin.

Projects which are to be displayed place emphasis on technical skills. Examples include murals, collages, posters and exhibitions. A selected group of patients plan and carry out the activity with the support or active assistance of the staff. Major benefits lie in the devolution of leadership and the making of decisions to the patients, as far as the ability of the group will allow. A sense of achievement can be based on the visual evidence of a successful outcome, and recognition can be gained from others when the finished work is displayed within the unit.

These benefits are not always experienced unless the activity is sensitively introduced and carried through. Therapists or helpers who have artistic ability or who are over-zealous may be tempted to dictate the finished result. An activity in which the ideas have been provided by a member of staff and an outline has been produced for patients to fill in does not demand greater creativity on the part of the patient than a repetitive industrial task. This is acceptable only if the patients experience genuine rewards in self-esteem from the technical merits of the finished product. On the other hand, a lack of guidance may lead to poor motivation and an experience of failure from the outset. Indiscriminate praise of patient's work, in this or any other context, can be counter-productive if not downright insulting. It is often appropriate to praise effort but to feign admiration for a product which is obviously incomplete, of poor quality or a disaster can imply low expectations of the patient's abilities. If every piece of work handed in by a student was returned by the supervisor or tutor marked 'super' then the poor student would be unable to apply standards or integrity to his own efforts.

Art which is destined for the bin concentrates on the benefits which can be gained through participation and disregards technical or artistic skills. Examples include imaginary journeys and meetings painted spontaneously on a large shared sheet of paper, imaginary battles and games played out on paper or blackboards between teams, and pictorial representations of immediate moods, problems or events. To maintain the spontaneity of such activities the sessions should be brief and undisrupted and materials should all be prepared in advance. The values are in the communication stimulated between members during the action and in providing opportunities for the expression of personal perceptions. Time should be allowed for discussion of the produced material at a level dictated by the participation of the patients. The willingness to express ideas through this kind of improvisation can be reduced by a therapist who is too quick to challenge or to interpret. 'Bin-art' as described here should not be confused with projective art in which analysis and personal exploration play a much greater part. Work with the majority of long-term patients is directed towards a simpler level of communication. Subjects should be chosen which encourage them to describe remembered events, to express awareness of their current situation and to indicate hopes or needs. The occupational therapist, in this context, is not seeking to identify unconscious material but to help patients to overcome difficulties in formulating and expressing ideas.

Modelling and sculpture

Making three-dimensional forms out of clay, papier mache or other materials can be a useful alternative to the media described above. Many people are hindered by a long-standing belief that they cannot draw, and relate two-dimensional art to failures and frustrations at school. Modelling materials may not have the same associations and are therefore more acceptable to many adults. Self-portraits, fantasies and animals are favourite starting points for those who are not wooed by the safety and anonymity of thumb pots and ash trays. A particular advantage of modelling in clay is that it is not difficult to achieve a result which is worthy of recognition. Simple sculpture or slab work can be very pleasing once glazed and fired. Working with other materials, a link can be formed with drama through the production of puppets, either individually or as a group project in preparation for a particular entertainment.

Group projects involving modelling and sculpture can be devised on a large scale and can involve a range of materials and levels of ability. Where the physical strength is available, projects involving brick, wood, clay, plaster, stone, or concrete may be more satisfying to adults than the use of washing-up liquid containers and egg boxes as constructional materials.

Creative writing

Many people experience, at some point in their lives, the pleasure which can be gained from writing, even if their peak experience is merely a particularly devastating letter of complaint to the local authority. Regular letter writing can be important to indviduals, as can be keeping a diary or writing down personal accounts of particular anxieties or pleasures. Although those who have received greater formal education may be more naturally inclined to write, this medium is in no way exclusive to this group. In fact they may find their creative attempts to be more greatly hindered by self-consciousness than people who have little experience of using the written word. By definition, anyone who is literate can write.

Creative writing does not have to mean poetry, although this is one of its most concise and interesting forms. A more acceptable introduction may be through descriptions of current events, letters and other factual records, gradually leading into experiemnts with fiction or fantasy. A magazine can be a useful vehicle for contributions by patients and staff, at the same time providing editorial and production responsibilities for individuals who need to extend their current roles.

Different ways of stimulating ideas can include story telling in a group or scripting a play for a particular range of human or puppet characters. The greatest resource that any individual has is his own previous experience. All memories are autobiographical material which could be written down given time and motivation, and every life is unique. There are a number of severely handicapped people who have produced fascinating personal histories.

Music

Making music and listening to music are activities which contain a strong emotional element. We often select music either to enhance or to change our current mood. Different types of music can serve to stimulate or to relax and are exploited for this reason, for example in shops and restaurants. Some people enjoy background music, some become oblivious to it after a time, and others find it an irritation and distraction. It should not be included as part of an environment for treatment without careful consideration of both its intention and who it is intended to please.

Listening to music can be used as a specific activity. It may help to improve an awareness of the environment and discrimination between tones and emotions. When short contrasting pieces are selected they can stimulate discussion about personal experiences and feelings. Some long-term patients apapear to have a very limited emotional range, that is they do not express either extremes of mood or fine variations in mood. This does not mean that they are not subject to the same fluctuations as others, but that they find emotional states difficult to identify and to communicate.

Music can be combined with other expressive forms such as movement or art. It can be easier to express abstract feelings through gestures or paintings than through words.

Making music has an infinite range of methods and of complexity. A very simple activity is to percuss different pieces of equipment, furniture, and implements in order to compare the sounds which they make in terms of volume, pitch and tone.

The human body can be made to produce a variety of rhythmic or interesting sounds including clapping, whistling, stamping, rubbing and slapping different parts. Orchestration of bodily functions is beyond the scope of this volume. The use of percussion instruments is of particular value both to the severely mentally handicapped and to the elderly and severely mentally infirm. A sense of rhythm is a very basic or primitive human ability and can both stimulate and reassure. Singing can be made as simple or demanding as abilities permit and can be used to enhance social harmony, concentration, confidence and even physical posture. Musical instruments can be used in a simple way to produce rhythms or easy tunes or they can become a sophisticated means of expression through improvisation, composition and performance.

Music can never be dismissed as being irrelevant or too difficult since it is a medium which can be adjusted to different purposes and levels of ability. Even the most unmusical therapist should consider ways in which the use of music could benefit patients and, when talent is called for, should call upon those who have it.

Remedial drama

There can be some confusion over the terms 'remedial drama', 'socio-drama' and 'psycho-drama' when these are applied to the use of drama within treatment. Although 'remedial drama' could be used to cover all three, it is possible to make general distinctions.

Remedial drama is the use of verbal and non-verbal exercises, games and improvisations to promote an awareness of oneself as an individual, an awareness of other people and the ability to express ideas.

Sociodrama consists of scenarios and role-playing exercises in order to simulate social situations, gain a better understanding of the dynamics involved in them and rehearse social behaviours which could be effective.

Psychodrama is a technique for exploring the dynamics and conflicts within one person's life. The individual acts out problematical situations within his life or relationships, using the other members of the group as he requires them. This is a method of treatment which in its pure form, is used only by those who have been specifically trained to do so.

In the context of long-term care, remedial drama is widely used with all groups of patients. Socio-drama is also relevant and is most appropriately included in a programme of training in social skills as described in Chapter 1.

Remedial drama does not have to imply an activity which is removed from reality. For patients whose grasp on reality is already weak such an emphasis would hardly be helpful. Exercises are chosen which express reality, in particular those which make a patient aware of his entire body including position, physical attitude, facial expression, gesture and voice. These exercises include physical movements such as curling up, stretching, reaching out and moving at different speeds. 'Mirroring' involves following and imitating the movements of a partner and requires awareness and concentration. Mime can involve concepts such as weight, texture, consistency and the size of different objects and materials. It can also illustrate different posturates and facial expressions and the meanings that are given to these. Other activities involve personal space, eye-contact and physical contact and contribute towards more effective communication. Improvising scenes and stories allows an individual to use his imagination within the controls of acting within a group and therefore needing to communicate his feelings and ideas to others.

Just as drama is used in schools to develop topics which are also being explored in other ways, remedial drama can be made relevant to other aspects of the patient's life. Current events, forthcoming changes and common difficulties can all form the nucleus of an idea which is developed as the theme of a drama session. For example, a group of severely mentally handicapped adults, about to go on a camping holiday, prepared for this experience through games and improvisations based on living out of doors.

Recreation

A patient's daily routine may include domestic duties, work, travel or specific treatment. These need to be balanced by recreation. For most people recreation includes organized activities such as sport, outings, holidays, clubs and social gatherings; and informal activities such as watching television, reading, talking, pursuing hobbies or taking exercise. The choice or recreational activities is normally related to age, sex, opportunity, ability and previous experience. In addition, an individual often chooses to do things in his spare time which fulfil needs unsatisfied by other parts of his routine. For example a sedentary or boring occupation may encourage someone to take up sporting or adventurous activities, an intellectually or physically demanding daily routine may create a need for relaxation or light entertainment.

Patients in hospital can be offered a variety of alternatives for the use of leisure time during the day, the evening or at weekends. These may include the provision of a television, games room, hobby area or organized social events. Such provisions are the joint responsibility of all those staff and volunteers who are committed to realizing the hospital as a place for living and not as a place of removal from life. Unfortunately many patients are unable to take advantage of such facilities due to a lack of social or cognitive abilities and difficulties in making personal decisions.

Patients who are not living in hospital may also experience problems in using their leisure time.

Those who are isolated, in particular the elderly, may not be able either to go out or arrange for people to visit them. Others may be unable to organize their lives to allow time or resources for enjoyment, or may have so much empty time that they cannot structure it into periods of routine tasks and recreation.

Although general recreation is not the sole preserve of

occupational therapy, recreational activities do have a place within treatment in certain circumstances. Firstly when organized sports, games, outings or events are an adjunct to training in communication, independence or social skills. Secondly, when a patient or client is unable to make choices or to organize his own leisure and therefore needs help to develop interests or to establish a routine.

Specific recreational activities such as table games, quizzes, pub games and discussions about current events may be used within a programme of treatment to increase motivation and orientation. This may be particularly important for very withdrawn patients or for the elderly. Those who have difficulty in concentrating for longer than a brief period may be helped to increase this span through activities which are enjoyable or mildly competitive.

The recreational needs of an individual cannot be completely satisfied by organisation imposed upon him by others. Such a contribution is an important part of caring, but an equal contribution is that of encouringing the patient, in gradual stages, to create his own opportunities.

Involvement of the community

Those who are not resident in hospital have more opportunity to use the same social facilities as other members of the community. Local streets, shops, pubs, clubs, leisure centres and parks are all places for normal social exchanges. Vulnerable people living at home, in group homes or in hostels are not segregated from the social world, although they may have to contend with suspicion or hostility from those who do not welcome them as a part of society.

People who live in hospital do not always have informal access to the same local facilities. A long separation from the world outside can make it increasingly difficult to return to it with confidence. Organized outings, involving large numbers of patients, to distant places of interest may serve useful functions but the maintenance of social contact within the community is not really one of them. Confidence and ability are more appropriately gained by the regular use of public transport, local shops and recreational facilities. Patients may need the support of a small group of fellow-patients or a member of staff, but they should not be easily identifiable by others as hospital patients due to their appearance or to obvious supervision by staff. A patient who is to be discharged after a long period in hospital needs to gain some experience of being on his own in crowded places, of planning his own evenings in clubs, pubs or cinemas and of finding his own way around the neighbourhood.

Some patients are too elderly, confused or frail to be able to leave the hospital. The community, therefore, has to be encouraged to come into the hospital. Volunteers, including school children, have a particularly important part to play. They can be regular visitors to a unit, form a special 'adoptive' link with one patient or provide planned entertainments to interrupt an otherwise unvaried routine.

Occupational therapists based in day centres are often involved in the running of clubs of 'ex-patients' who need background social support and an informal access to professional help in times of stress. As psychiatric treatment for all groups of patients becomes more centred in the community, and as the large distant hospitals are phased out in favour of smaller local units within district general hospitals, such co-ordinating roles will become even more important. Treating people within the context of their own social environment helps to eliminate problems arising from an abnormal society and the need to simulate social settings and opportunities. It also means involving many more people within a programme of treatment and enlisting the sympathy and participation of members of the community.

PERSONAL ACTIVITIES

Looking after oneself and one's immediate environment does not rely only on the cognitive and physical ability to acquire skills. One needs to be motivated by a sense of personal identity which involves an awareness of other people's responses, and a standard of physical comfort and integrity. It is also necessary to have free access to the facilities which allow one to practise autonomy without having to be dependent on the controls or routines of others.

Personal care

Long-term patients can sometimes be identified, in the vicinity of treatment units or hospitals, by their physical appearance. Typical features include a poor physical posture, a shuffling or slow gait, ill-fitting or inappropriate clothing and unfashionable hairstyles. Clients living in the community do not totally avoid such problems, although their clothing does escape the punishing effects of hospital laundries.

The reasons for people looking a bit odd are various, but fall into two main categories. Firstly there is the patient's lack of awareness or concern about his personal presentation, and secondly there are the circumstances which make him dependent on others for the way that he looks. Obviously these two are closely connected. The patient's own lack of concern may be based on his having become accustomed to his clothing being provided, and by responsibility for his personal hygiene having been assumed by others.

Patients who appear well-dressed and cared for may owe this to a conscientious charge nurse or to the intervention of members of his family or support services. The problems facing most patients are those of relearning personal skills and regaining the roles and responsibilities of a physically independent person.

The care of the body includes care of hair, skin, nails, and teeth and general cleanliness and personal enhancement. Men need to be able to shave and women, of child-bearing age, to manage menstruation.

Responsibility for clothing includes choice and purchase, storage, correct laundering and basic repairs.

Training in these matters should develop not only the skills required to carry out each task but also discretion, that is, a knowledge of when to carry them out and what equipment or materials to use. Within hospitals the patient's use of discretion is controlled by whether he can select and own his own soap, toothpaste, shampoo and so forth and whether he can be given free access to washing and laundry facilities.

A patient may learn to use, for example, washing machines and hairdriers, or to manicure nails or use cosmetics, within the occupational therapy department. According to the ability of the patient, or the complexity of the task, teaching may be broken down into stages, be repeated at intervals or be covered in a single session. The success of any such teaching is dependent on the patient's opportunity to rehearse the behaviour and integrate it within his own routine. For this reason occupational therapists and nurses need to work in close collaboration to provide consistent expectation of, and opportunities for, the patient.

Sex can be included under the general heading of personal care although most people would regard it as a social activity. Some, of course, may consider it to be a household task or even a form of employment. Indecent exposure and public masturbation are, however, personally untidy and offensive to others and can therefore be discouraged on the same grounds that an awareness of, and pride in, personal appearance are encouraged.

Promiscuity is usually defined by someone who is outside the relationship in question. It is impossible to generalize theoretically about whether people should have sexual intercourse or not and it may be more important to consider where they can reasonably do so and whether any undesirable consequences can be avoided. In hospitals, hostels and some group homes, privacy is not easy to find. Patients who are living at home with families may also experience restrictions or disapproval in this respect although their independence is being actively encouraged in other ways.

The provision of sexual opportunities may not be the direct function of an occupational therapist, but teaching the use of contraceptives is often a necessary part of a programme in personal care. Since other skills are taught in simple terms or at a level appropriate to the patient's ability, contraception should be no exception. A basic understanding of why protection is needed does not have to involve an intense study of anatomical diagrams and complex terminology, just as when learning to use a washing machine, one needs to know what to do and when to do it to ensure effectiveness rather than absorb the entire wiring and plumbing system.

Food

An independent person needs to be able to plan a balanced

diet, to buy provisions, store them correctly, prepare meals or drinks and maintain a reasonably hygienic kitchen. This may sound easy but in fact involves a complex range of abilities.

Planning does not have to involve detailed knowledge of vitamins, minerals and calorific values. Most people survive, and most families are raised, on a mixture of common sense and tradition. The body often expresses its own specific needs through an appetite for particular types of food. It is useful to know that protein can be obtained from meat, fish, eggs, cheese, pulses and, in smaller quantities, from a range of other foods. Fruit and green vegetables form an important part of the diet and so does a regular input of bulk or roughage. One rarely needs to advise people to include carbohydrates in their diet since foods containing these are often already being consumed to excess. This may seem oversimplified but one should relate the need for knowledge to healthy living and not to theoretical examinations in nutrition. A patient who has special dietary needs will simply require deeper understanding. People at special risk include the schizophrenic who is abnormally indiscriminate in his diet and the elderly who may neglect themselves, not through lack of experience but through confusion or lack of volition.

Buying food is a particular problem for the single person. 'Convenience foods' packaged in single portion are comparatively expensive but it can be difficult to find fresh foods which can be purchased in irregularly small quantities. Supermarkets tend to package meat and vegetables to suit families, and small shops willing to sell, for example, one onion and three sausages may have to offset their overheads in higher prices. To produce regular meals certain basic stocks of dried and tinned foods are essential, together with a regular supply of milk, beverages and condiments. The patient who is providing his own meals needs to know what basic supplies to have in stock and what food must be bought fresh each week.

Storing food correctly is essential to maintaining one's own physical health. Stale cornflakes and wizened fruit may be quite harmless but elderly meat and repeatedly reheated meals can have some nasty effects. Knowledge of how to keep food wholesome involves that of proper conditions and temperatures, the defrosting of refrigerators and when not to take risks.

Cooking can be as simple or as complex as the individual chooses. It may be more relevant to teach the intelligent use of prepared or 'convenience' foods than to spend time practising the management of fresh meat and vegetables. The specific tasks given emphasis by the occupational therapist will depend on the patient's intended future environment. Some people need only to be able to make a cup of tea or to prepare the occasional snack, others must learn sufficient to provide themselves with a total and varied diet.

Safety and hygiene must be considered within a programme of teaching. The dangers of mishandled gas or electricity may be the factor preventing an irresponsible person from living an unsupervised life. Grubby utensils may not be as dramatically hazardous as blazing chip-pans but a patient who is likely to produce either may be a potential danger to himself or to others.

Household tasks

Outside the kitchen many tasks have to be accomplished in order to maintain a standard of safety and comfort.

General order involves routine activities such as making beds, changing sheets, emptying ashtrays and airing rooms. Those who can maintain domestic order are not merely people who have learned faithfully to follow a routine but are people who are aware of their environment. Staff can be over-efficient in adjusting temperature, ventilation and light on behalf of patients, without involving them in these minor decisions. This can encourage individuals to become unaware of their immediate environment and ultimately less able to control it.

Many new products and pieces of equipment are now available to make household tasks easier, but their variety can cause additional confusion and expense. Patients should be encouraged to discuss the relative merits of aerosol polishes, liquid cleansers, abrasives and so forth. Persuasive advertising can mislead one into believing that a different product is required for the successful completion of every cleaning process.

Patients who are moving away from hospital need to know, for example, when to change the paper bag inside vacuum cleaners, the sponge head on mops or the window cleaner if he proves to be a crook. Simple household duties include changing defunct light-bulbs for new ones of the correct wattage, replacing fuses and batteries and keeping pilot flames alight, as well as routine cleaning. It is important to know what jobs should be tackled and what situations require outside help or advice. Running a home involves the ability to solve problems and to use appropriate resources. The style in which a patient wishes to live is his own decision but should not be the consequence of inability or lack of access to help.

Personal administration

Organisational and financial aspects of living can be very complicated. Even an otherwise healthy individual can become bewildered by the necessity to balance income and expenditure, to interpret official forms and commercial advertising and both to claim his benefits from and pay his dues to different government departments.

Budgeting can be considered, and taught, on different levels. Simple budgeting is the ability to plan expenditure in one context only, for example food, with a fixed daily or weekly sum of money to spend. This is the simplest financial task to be included in a programme of rehabilitation. Complex budgeting involves the allocation of money, from a predetermined sum, to different purposes. For example the weekly income may be divided into money for food, rent, electricity, recreation, clothing, household sundries and savings. This is the next stage in acquiring the ability to handle money and involves planning ahead in each of the separate 'accounts'. Total control of finances is the final stage and includes responsibility for income. This involves claiming all benefits to which one is entitled, managing a bank or post office savings account, filling in tax forms in relation to earnings and forecasting future needs.

Different methods of payment exist for power bills, rates, television licences, fares for daily transport and major purchases. Some are based on spreading payments over a period of time through instalments or special savings stamps. Others, for example bus, underground and train fares, involve payment in advance in order to benefit from special rates.

Appeals from charities and advertising material make up a proportion of everyone's daily post. It is necessary to discriminate between these and official communications and to deal with unsolicited gifts which arrive with optional bills for payments or inducements to enter competitions. Advertisements in the press which promise solutions to every imaginable physical, psychological or sensory deficit can find easy prey in those who are disabled, anxious or who have a low self-esteem.

A programme of learning which is based on predictable demands will always be caught out sooner or later. One cannot prepare an individual to meet every situation which might later present itself. The next bang on the door could be a salesman, a missionary, a complaining neighbour or the man from the gas board. All teaching should be based on the patient identifying and increasing his own abilities, being able to work through problems systematically and knowing when and where assistance should be sought.

Elderly people who are living alone may find personal administration particularly difficult and may extend an otherwise useful degree of suspicion to include advances from helpful agencies or governmental departments. The most important part of learning may be to identify at least one person who is considered trustworthy, whether a member of the family, social services department or local community, who can help to sort out problems as they arise.

WORK AND CONSTRUCTIVE ACTIVITIES

The activities grouped together in this section all have some tangible reward or result. Work, on an industrial production line or within another environment which has recognisable parallels in open employment, is the most significant.

Hamilton & Salmon (1962) showed 20 years ago that industrial therapy compared favourably with occupational therapy in terms of its capacity to improve a patient's social competence and clinical state. The greater benefits appeared to arise from both the presence of a financial reward and from working within a structured and male-dominated environment on a socially acceptable task. This does not mean that the majority of occupational therapists should change their professional philosophy and their sex but that we should pay particular attention to the benefits which can be gained through providing quasi-industrial work. Status and self-esteem are socially embedded in productive tasks, employment and wages. However, the above study was carried out with male chronic schizophrenic patients of employable age. The problems presented by the long-term psychiatric population as a whole are more diverse. The overwhelming majority of patients are unlikely to return to open employment due either to their age or to the shortage of jobs available. Rehabilitation cannot be based on the premise that useful employment is a normal expectation and that status and success are measurable only in terms of wages. The reality is that we rehabilitate the majority of patients for either a retired life-style or coping with unemployment. This involves finding satisfaction in alternative activities and being able to structure a routine around hobbies, interests, voluntary work and social contacts.

Industrial work

The environmental considerations in using industrial work were considered in Chapter 9. Tasks should be realistic, structured and related to financial reward. The discipline which accompanies efficient production contributes to the sense of identity experienced by a patient and the development of his role as a 'worker'.

Problems can arise if pressure on the time allowed for the completion of contract work redirects the concerns of the staff towards the contract rather than towards the patients. Suitable tasks can be difficult to secure and the patients may therefore be employed below their own level of capability or with insufficient variety.

In some regions or units the organization of industrial work is one of the responsibilities of the occupational therapy department. In others, this function is fulfilled by nurses or by workshop managers. Providing that the workshop is run effectively, and that the most appropriate patients are referred for this form of activity, then semi-professional territorial arguments are unwarranted. Certain ethical problems arise, such as whether patients shold 'retire' from therapeutic work at the age of 65, raise further problems. Work ceases to be therapeutic when the patient's happiness and self-esteem become invested in it to the exclusion of alternatives.

Heavy workshops

However strong the intellectual arguments for sexual equality in all spheres of life, many activities carry an implication of sexual identity. It is true that many men enjoy tapestry and many women enjoy bricklaying but one cannot force such choices on any individual. Part of the provision of occupational therapy departments is the inclusion of activities such as woodwork, metalwork and building. More men than women may benefit from such activities, particularly if the organisation and teaching is placed in the hands of a male member of staff. Projects undertaken in workshops include both fine work by individuals and projects involving groups of patients, such as furniture making, upholstery or producing equipment for the disabled. The atmosphere in such workshops should be purposeful and should encourage co-operation between individuals. Physically strenuous activities increase tolerance to both fatigue and noise and also channel energy in a constructive way. If high standards of work are expected, skills in handling tools can be gained and satisfaction in the finished result justified.

Light workshops

'Light' work includes printing, simple assembly, typing, filing and any other activity which is productive but not physically strenuous. Many such tasks require a high degree of cognitive ability. Printing is a useful example since it is a process which can be divided into tasks of varying complexity from simply slotting paper into a press and pulling a handle, to designing and setting up a specified order. The management of a printing unit also involves receiving orders, preparing estimates, establishing priorities in production, controlling quality and invoicing clients. Printing can therefore provide a progressive programme of activities for an indvidual and be graded to almost any level of ability.

Clerical work, such as filing, typing, book-keeping and stock control also provides varying degrees of intellectual demand and responsibility. Such tasks may be related to the needs of the unit, such as by producing magazines or news-sheets, or by contributing to the administration through keeping records of attendance, payment or materials.

Involvement in this range of activities may be preparatory to further training or employment, but equally may provide a satisfying routine which develops potential through the acquisition of skills and a sense of being of value.

Crafts

Handwork such as stool-seating, canework, weaving, sewing and toymaking has been traditionally associated with occupational therapy. In more recent years the profession has developed alternative techniques in order to meet a wider range of needs. Qualified therapists no longer devote time to knitting, knotting, netting or stuffing rabbits. Although it takes a long time for skills to evolve and for roles to develop, it takes even longer for such changes to be recognized by colleagues, clients and the general public. This has caused some impatience and frustration within the profession and a more vehement rejection of crafts than is necessarily warranted.

When crafts are used specifically to increase abilities to make decisions, to persevere, to handle tools, to concentrate, to share responsibility with others, or for any other predetermined purpose, they remain most useful media for treatment. A resurgence of national interest in the traditional crafts has, in recent years, helped to re-establish their social acceptability. If each process is analysed and selected, on the basis of its component qualities or demands, as being useful to the treatment of an individual patient then craftwork has considerable future potential.

Poor use of craftwork can be seen in departments where there is an inadequate ratio of therapists to patients and where traditions in treatment have been continued without evaluation. Activities in such an environment may achieve little beyond the filling of time.

There is a need to distinguish between diversional activity, which can be instigated by occupational therapists but carried out by craft teachers or volunteers, and programmes of treatment in which crafts are used to develop specific abilities or responsibilities.

Gardening and husbandry

Growing plants and looking after animals are activities with unique properties. Without overstating the case, each places miracles within the reach of otherwise incapacitated mortals. A rural and agricultural environment used to provide a tolerant and creative environment for the less able and this tradition was carried on when large asylums had their own farmland and were essentially self-supporting. However, many such acres have now been sold to, and built over by, developers and union control of labour has thrived on the platform of neither excluding the workforce nor exploiting the patients. The result of all this progress is known as horticultural therapy and attempts to re-unite the patient with pre-industrial pleasures.

Activities which can be used range through caring for greenhouses, domestic gardening, market gardening and growing field crops. The care of animals can be as simple as keeping a budgerigar or as ambitious as running a herd of cattle. Relationships with animals are different from relationships with people. Animals are essentially honest, offer devotion without unjustified criticism and do not answer back. They also respect one's confidence and respond through behaviour rather than through additions to medical records.

Plants and animals can give a patient the experience of being in control, providing he attends to their needs. In growing, being productive and dying they present a microcosm of life in all its phases and an acceptance of each.

BIBLIOGRAPHY

Hamilton V, Salmon P 1962 Psychological changes in chronic schizophrenics following differential activity programmes. Journal of Mental Science 108:455, 505–520
Hopkins H L, Smith H D (eds) 1978 Willard and Spackman's occupational therapy, 5th edn. J B Lippincott, Philadelphia
Llorens L A 1976 Applications of developmental theory for health and rehabilitation. American Occupational Therapy Association

RECOMMENDED READING

Alvin J 1966 Music therapy. John Baker, London
Bennett D 1970 The value of work in psychiatric rehabilitation. Social Psychiatry 5: 224–230
Brandes D, Phillips The gamesters handbook. Hutchinson, London
Carver V, Liddiard P 1978 An ageing population. Hodder and Stoughton, Sevenoaks. In association with the Open University Press
Jennings S 1973 Remedial drama. Pitman, London
Jennings S (ed) 1975 Creative therapy. Pitman, London
Kramer D 1977 Art as therapy with children. Schoken Books, New York
Langley D M, Langley G E 1983 Dramatherapy and psychiatry. Croom Helm, London
Liberman R P et al 1975 Personal effectiveness. Research Press, Illinois
Pavey D 1979 Art based games. Methuen, London
Priestly P et al 1978 Social skills and personal problem solving. Tavistock, London
Remocker A J, Storch E T 1987 Action speaks louder, 4th edn. Churchill Livingstone, Edinburgh
Stevens J O 1971 Awareness: exploring, experimenting, experiencing. Real People
Way B 1967 Development through drama. Longman, London
Warren B 1984 Using the creative arts in therapy. Croom Helm, London
Whelan E, Speake B 1979 Learning to cope. Souvenir Press, London

11

Community care

INTRODUCTION

The time will come when 'community care' loses its relevance as the title for a separate chapter. The present inclusion reflects current concerns within the history of psychiatry, a conscious movement away from a past system of care towards a revised social context. In this sense we are not discovering a new era but are rather bringing to a close an old one. The medically prescribed removal of psychiatrically impaired people from the community has been a social phase dominating only a couple of centuries. Within this time span two particular phenomena are notable, one medical and one social. Recently the scientific study of mental disorders has made spectacular strides, including the advent of powerful psychotrophic drugs, the rise of behaviouralism and the systematisation of theories of personality and psychotherapy. Secondly, society has learned in general to do without the irregularities and inconveniences of its psychologically disordered members. The possibility, and then desirability, of removing the inadequate and the inconvenient has enabled us to exclude a high proportion of mentally handicapped, behaviourally disturbed and socially deteriorating people from patterns of social life which are accepted as being normal. Naturally, tolerance to extremes of need has tended to reduce, producing a narrowed *public* view of acceptable social performance. However, at the same time and perhaps as a reaction to this, there has been a rising *private* concern for the rights of disabled people. This has resulted in individuals or families being less inclined to conceal mental health problems and in corporate activities such as those of MIND, MENCAP, the Schizophrenia Fellowship and other client-based service or pressure groups.

The current emphasis in community care centres on two major issues: the discharge of long-term patients after appropriate rehabilitation and the positive choice to treat new referrals without unnecessary recourse to institutional care. Both of these concerns involve the provision of a comprehensive service comprising relevant staff and facilities for both treatment and support. The policy of rehabilitating and resettling long-term patients has followed the obvious pattern of starting with the most able and working through the strata of functional ability. This stratification has been expedient for rehabilitation teams as clients of roughly equivalent capabilities have been selected for retraining at the appropriate level. Outside hospitals, those services which have been provided have been oriented towards the needs of the recently discharged groups. In some areas this has resulted in a reactive pattern of community services. It is interesting to speculate on the structure of support which would have been perceived as being necessary had the rehabilition of long-term patients been conceived in a different way, involving from the outset, mixed levels of ability.

Just as services have had to expand to meet the needs of the different strata of people emerging from long-term institutional care, they have also had to extend to cater for those being treated as short-term admissions or not admitted at all. Outpatient clinics and 'drop-in' centres are clearly only the tip of the iceberg. Full-or part-time day care and individual support or therapy may be necessary for clients and, of equal importance, support and guidance for families and friends who may be the willing or less willing full-time carers.

At the time of writing there is considerable variation in the provision for long-term clients in different geographical locations. There are fears that the policies underlying community care may be damaging to the quality of clients' lives when the rate of discharge is not equalled by a commitment to provide alternative sources of daytime care, suitable accommodation or long-term social support. There are also instances of sound, committed and well integrated systems providing treatment and care. A basic text such as this does not seek to applaud or to condemn current initiatives. Its task is to identify problems, establish principles and to suggest directions for professional activity. The principles governing the design of occupational therapy are the same as those applied within institutionally based treatment. The fundamental tasks of assessment, selection of therapeutic mode, goal setting, programme planning and evaluation are still performed. Operating outside a hospital does not permit a therapist to abandon theoretically sound and practically orientated methods of practice in favour of generalised multi-professional muddle. It does provide a real and changing climate within which intervention can have on immediate impact on the client. There are many clear advantages in working within an environment which is not simulated to be life-like but is life.

PROVISIONS WITHIN THE COMMUNITY

Organisation

It has already been acknowledged that facilities for care in the community vary from one area to another. The evolution of a comprehensive service tends to be subject to perceived need, to available funding and to the motivation of professional staff and other interested people. The following information is gleaned from current developments in different parts of the United Kingdom. An effective system may not include all of the provisions described, but is constructed from elements selected for their relevance to the local situation.

A significant factor in the evolution of services is the source and control of money. A move from institutional to community care involves some shifting of financial responsibility from the Health Service to Local Authorities. Adjustments in the organisation of public expenditure need to be carefully planned and involve a gradual process which must remain in parallel with the reduction in the number of people receiving institutional care. The partnership between the Health Service and the Social Services has been cemented by the creation of Joint Consultative Committees. These have been statutory committees of each Health Authority since the re-organisation of the Health Service in 1974. The membership includes representation from the Social Services Authorities. The real action, however, is usually found at the next level down, the Joint Care Planning Teams. The membership of these includes the senior officers from the represented bodies. Representatives can also be co-opted from voluntary bodies.

These Joint Care Planning Teams give rise, in their turn, to a further level of sub-groups: for example the 'joint care co-ordinating groups' at district level. Representatives from Housing Associations are often involved at this level, if not within the Planning Team itself. The life-blood of this structure is 'Joint Finance', money in the Health Authority's allocation from central Government which is available to initiatives within the community. It makes sense for Health Authorities to transfer some of their funds to support community projects where these meet the service objectives more effectively than could be achieved through direct expenditure. Joint funding is not intended to be a permanent financial arrangement but enables the development of new services. Once established these need long-term support through the transfer of central funds. An important point is that joint finance is not limited to Health and Social Service initiatives but is available to voluntary organisations, Housing Associations and individual projects. This flexibility has made possible a wide variety of pilot schemes involving long-stay hostels, half-way houses, peripatetic rehabilitation support teams, activity centres and other forms of day care. Information on what is happening and where becomes out of date or incomplete within a short space of time. Sources of information about current projects are therefore given at the end of this chapter.

Individual elements

The environments and services described here do not constitute an exhaustive list of all projects in which occupational therapists may have involvement. They are selected for their relevance to the support of long-term patients.

The core and cluster concept

The model proposes a 'cluster' or network of houses or services which all relate to a central or 'core' unit. The core unit is essentially an administrative centre which co-ordinates the service to each client, it may also provide a base for the Community Mental Health Team. Individual units within the network or 'cluster' are usually houses acquired for a small number of clients who are living together. The system may also embrace individuals living on their own, in lodgings or with families. The effectiveness of this model is reliant on its flexibility. Support for each unit can be varied from 24-hour coverage to periodical visits and can be increased or decreased according to the needs of any individual client. Staff time, as a core resource, can be allocated to make the maximum and most economical use of skills. Clients who gain in independence will experience a gradual withdrawal of support rather than being disrupted by a move to a less supported environment.

Half-way houses

These are now a well-established feature of programmes of rehabilitation. Many of the original units were established within the grounds of a hospital or not too far away. It is, however, more important that they are situated close to resources within the community. A place in a 'half-way house' should provide a person with opportunities to practise domestic, personal and social skills but still allow him access to support or help from familiar members of staff. He may be spending the daytime in hospital-based treatment or work activities; alternatively he may be working outside the hospital or attending a day centre. Residence in a half-way house is intended to be a temporary phase preceding full resettlement. During this phase an occupational therapist would expect to maintain close contact and to continue the teaching of basic skills.

Group homes

These often provide a first home for groups of patients discharged together from hospital. Such groups may have worked through a programme of rehabilitation together and may be selected for their compatibility or their complementary skills. The permanence of such a group depends largely on their continuing to share abilities and interests. Those more capable or more inclined to be solitary may naturally gravitate to a more independent life-style. Living together in a group brings social pressures as well as advantages and individuals continue to change. The population of a group home is therefore likely to be fluid, but such an environment can provide a realistic environment for a client over an extended period. Where the core and cluster model is being used the group home will receive support from the core unit.

Hostels

A hostel can provide structures and routines for those who are unable to establish these for themselves. They offer, to the more vulnerable or dependent, support and protection from exploitation or unkindness as well as a residential base. Most hostels provide social rather than medical care but employ staff who will seek, on the patients' behalf, any additional help that they may need. Residents are usually expected to maintain their domestic skills by helping to run the hostel. During the day they may be in sheltered or open employment or attending a day unit. Problems can be created by hostels that are closed during the day when other facilities are inadequate or non-existing.

Day centres

These may be orientated towards work, social contact, individually planned programmes or group work. Part of their purpose is to provide a focus or routine for unemployed and vulnerable people living in the community and to relieve the pressures on family carers. The occupational therapists' contribution is often to provide specific training in domestic or work activities or social skills, or to assess and treat individual behavioural problems. It is important that clients are able to organise their own attendance at a day centre which may involve the use of local transport. In rural areas, and in some dense city conurbations, this can involve difficulties and distances that prove too great. Travelling day units have therefore evolved which can move each day to a different location and provide a once or twice weekly service to clients. Such mobile services are able to make use of a variety of public or private buildings central to small towns or residential areas.

Activity centres

These differ from day centres in that they do not offer treatment to selected clients but provide opportunities for any individual to use if he wants to. Some such centres have developed within hospitals and are open to in-patients and 'ex-patients' alike, others are situated as informal community resources. Those attending prescribe their own activities, within the resources that the centre can offer, and wherever possible participate in day-to-day management.

Social clubs and informal groups

Social clubs and informal or 'self-help' groups can be established as an adjunct to day-care. Those who have established a normal routine of independent living may still want contacts to be maintained as a safety net. These organisations allow access to others who have shared similar problems in the past, and to professional help in times of difficulty. For the elderly, or for others who may be experiencing a relatively isolated life-style, attending a club or group may provide a social focus.

THE OCCUPATIONAL THERAPIST IN THE COMMUNITY

Different patterns of provision which have emerged in different places provide a range of contexts in which occupational therapists may be employed. Some are based within Social Service teams and either have a case-load of disabled clients or particular responsibilities for day centres or support units run by Social Service Departments. Others may be employed by the Health Service and may be based in day hospitals or centres, in hospitals from which they make therapeutic excursions, or attached to health centres. Private organisations and charities may employ occupational therapists within residential units, day care facilities or in advisory or training capacities. The previous section indicated the range of environments in which a therapist may work, irrespective of the employer. Although the organisational structure has a major influence on the tasks performed there are a number of basic roles which are usually involved. These include providing specific programmes of treatment for individuals or groups, being a resource or catalyst to promote activity, providing optimum environments for long-term support and working effectively as a member of a team.

Providing specific treatment

Training in practical skills, which may have formed a major part in the pre-discharge programme, must often be continued for some time after resettlement. If a patient is discharged to a hostel or to other supervised accommodation he may not be required to put skills to immediate use and may forget, or lose confidence, in those he has acquired. Clients who have remained in the care of their own families or social networks may also be unskilled in personal and domestic tasks. This may only become identified as a problem when the family becomes stressed or when a move to a more independent life-style is being considered. A third group of clients may, through prolonged anxiety, depression or other problems, have ceased to use the skills which they possess. In these circumstances the problem is usually a loss of confidence coupled with difficulties in structuring time. Practical work with all these people can be undertaken either in suitably equipped day units or in their own homes. The latter is often more effective although it may preclude the benefits of working in small groups. Individual programmes should be designed in direct relationship with current and future needs. Those living in close contact with the client should have a detailed knowledge of the programme so that they can be active in encouraging the rehearsal of skills.

The teaching of community skills, such as using shops, post offices, benefits offices and leisure facilities, is the logical extension of a domestic programme. Every opportunity should be taken to help clients to develop organisational skills in structuring their own use of time. Initially this may require detailed help in the time-tabling of each day and the setting of personal goals. It is important to be aware of the natural 'pace' of each individual since routines which attempt too much or too little are self defeating.

Training in social skills can be continued or introduced to groups in the community with particular benefits being derived from being able to set tasks or to rehearse skills under genuine conditions. Any other form of treatment used within institutions can be applied in day units, hostels or private homes. It must be noted, when a behavioural model is being used, that a wide range of people are in daily contact with the client. Time must be given to explaining exactly what is happening and to encouraging significant people to collaborate with the programme.

Promoting activity

Working on the general principle that one hour's positive and self-motivated activity on the part of a client can be worth up to 100 hours on the part of the therapist, an essential role is that of 'catalyst'. The therapist should be exceptionally well informed about all local facilities and events. This knowledge should not be limited to statutory and voluntary provisions for the disadvantaged but should extend over the locality. Aim to be a comprehensive social encyclopaedia of the physical, recreational, cultural and spiritual life of the community. Encourage clients to become involved in existing activities, at first accompanied and later on their own. Early contact with the use of these resources tends to be made in organised groups. This may be for financial reasons, for ease of planning and supervision and to give clients peer-group support. However, it is seldom a good idea to develop a routine of large group outings to parks, exhibitions, sports centres or entertainments. The general public are invaded rather than educated and the clients retain a segregated identity. Whenever four staff are accompanying twelve patients the reasons for such an arrangement should have been clearly identified. Two, three or four separate ventures may be a great deal more beneficial for all concerned with the exception of the staff.

Social skills training and social activities can be effective in increasing skills, confidence and knowledge of resources, but they do not necessarily lead to a more gregarious life-style. Those clients who prefer to be solitary may have learned to restrict social contact to a level which they find both healthy and conducive. This requires a therapist to be imaginative in promoting activities which add an interest and structure to daily living but which are not personally invasive.

'Self-help' groups are recognised as a valuable source of support and identity for a variety of clients living in the community. Once in existence they provide an immediate reference group for new members who in turn may benefit from being able to assist others. However self-perpetuating these may be, help is required in the early stages to set them up and to establish their initial membership and activities. The organisation of such a group will vary according to its selective membership; whether they are depressed and unemployed men, isolated mothers, group home dwellers, retired single people, parents of mentally handicapped children, carers for elderly relatives or hippophobic horse-dealers. However, since the intention is for the group to maintain itself with only intermittent professional involvement a few principles can be generalised.

1. The time and place of meetings should be regular, widely known and not subject to alteration at short notice.
2. There should be a balance between time devoted to discussion and time given to planned activity. Discussion alone tends to deteriorate into negative grumbles. Activity serves to unite the membership in positive co-operation. Activity without discussion does not contribute to the specific needs of the membership.
3. Leadership should not be vested in one member for too long but should rotate as far as possible among the members.
4. The outside instigator of the group should retain an interest in its work and help it to survive 'low' patches or specific problems.

The therapist should also be concerned in promoting activity in the sphere of public involvment. Part of this process involves providing information about mental health and alerting people to the related problems and needs. Voluntary bodies, youth groups and individuals who are made aware of exactly how they can help will often be happy to do so. Their contribution may be practical, such as fund-raising or house decorating, or personal such as befriending individual clients. The social life of a disturbed or disabled person has to rely on formal or informal volunteers, at least until he is able to initiate and maintain his own social network.

Enabling others to act, whether they are clients, volunteers or colleagues, can best be achieved by providing a conducive environment. Refer back at this stage to Chapter 9 which outlines some of the principles involved. Any therapeutic environment has two components, physical features and prevailing attitudes. Physical features of day units, hostels, group homes or any other place of care should include all the comforts and opportunities of well-established family home. Think about a familiar home environment which provides both security and creative opportunities. What are its attributes beyond a kitchen and living space? A garden? A greenhouse? A workshop? Evidence of games, hobbies, current enthusiasms and projects? Even a dedicated musician would find a room full of low tables and an upright piano a poor source of inspiration. Prevailing attitudes should encourge but not bully people, competent and enthusiastic therapists fail at the point where their qualities overwhelm others or make them feel comparatively helpless.

Working within a team

In any working environment the extent to which professional roles can overlap, before anxiety over identity is invoked, is dependent on individual relationships. Smaller units do, however, tend to involve greater numerical equality between the occupational groups. A combination of good working relationships and equal respresentation should allow better teamwork than institutional power politics and hierarchies sometimes allow. Within the community a wider range of people may be actively involved in both treatment and maintenance. For example, those in close contact with one client may include his family, friends, voluntary workers, neighbours, psychiatrist, general practitioner, psychologist, occupational therapist, community psychiatric nurse, social worker, landlord, clergyman, solicitor and as many others as circumstances have involved. Many of these people are unlikely to meet, and have little knowledge of each other's involvement.

Regular case conferences play an important role in co-ordinating and evaluating progress. These tend to be restricted to 'professional' members of the team and are alarmingly expensive. It is therefore essential both to represent the views and contribution of those not present and to be thorough in preparation so that time is used productively. In many areas a key worker scheme is in operation. This member of the team takes responsibility for co-ordinating the contributions that others make to the care of a client and his family. The key worker also ensures that every individual involved has access to relevant information. It is also helpful to the client, and to those close to him, to have a designated person to contact when the need arises.

THE INSTITUTION WITHIN THE COMMUNITY

Despite professional or public resolve to rehabilitate long-stay patients, or to care for new referrals with minimum recourse to admission, psychiatric institutions continue to exist. They are populated by residual long-term patients, who may be multiply handicapped or aging, and by the 'new long-stay' group. There are three major reasons for continuing institutional care. The first is the severity of the condition and its resistance to available treatment. The second is the lack of social support for elderly or disturbed family members, due not always to lack of concern but to resources, relationships and to diverse commitments. The third is the choice made by the client who may have a strong preference for a protected and dependent life-style.

Psychiatric hospitals have almost halved their population over the last 30 years, however, since they continue to play a major part within the service, it is relevant to discuss their future role. Are they to be asylums in the sense of escape and protection from society? Are they to be integrated and developed as a resource within a coherent strategy for psychiatric care? To what extent do their stigmatised histories interfere with realistic plans for the future?

The institution as a social resource

In our concern to discharge patients from hospital and to resettle them in the community, public resources have figured significantly within programmes of treatment. Local parks, the post office, shops, libraries and facilities for sport and entertainment all become involved. There are a wide range of possibilities because society has gradually equipped itself with an extensive network of services to provide health care, education and leisure activities. When many of the large psychiatric hospitals were built these were deliberately placed outside centres of population and some of them remain in inconvenient or isolated positions. Where cities have expanded to *enclose* the institutions they have not necessarily *included* them within the social network except as a source of employment. It is this exclusion of institutions from the community that has contributed to concepts such as the 'return of patients to the community' and providing 'facilities for community care'. In the long-term, however, this is not going to be enough. The psychiatric institution, as an excluded place of removal from society, also needs to be rehabilitated back into the community. This is not an easy task, frequently identified problems include the rigid and hierarchical attitudes of staff and the need to educate the public. Educating the public involves providing information about the problems and needs created by psychiatric disorders, providing reassurance about possible dangerous or anti-social behaviour, and producing miraculously changed attitudes which lead to genuine welcome, tolerance and concern. The last one is a bit difficult to manage, as Douglas Bennett commented back in 1979: '. . . it is assumed that the community is therapeutic and really cares, although no source is quoted for this assumption. As a result the possibility that the community could not care is not discussed.' It is, of course individuals who care. When enough individuals care the community acts. The community must act positively in relation to institutions if they are to be drawn back into society.

In simple terms, to promote genuine 'community care' we have to create a flow in two directions; an outward move of patients from the institution to the community and an inward flow of healthy people from the community into the institution — so that it no longer remains an excluded place. The inward flow is essential to destigmatise the institution and to reduce the isolation and rejection of those in its care. The remainder of this book is about the rehabilitation of patients, the outward flow. The following comments are about the rehabilitation of the institution which includes the reorientation of staff and the promotion of the inward flow. There is work here for a whole army of imaginative occupational therapists.

One of the central problems is that psychiatric hospitals have traditionally offered only one public service, the accommodation and treatment of socially embarassing people. This is perfectly sensible but it does not motivate general public participation. Although some very good voluntary schemes exist, which involve visits from school children, organisations or individuals, those involved are pre-selected by altruism, social awareness or the need for occupation or recognition. They are more usually providers of service than consumers. If the hospital is the best local source of a desirable commodity or facility then people of greater variety and in larger numbers start to be involved and the concept of integration becomes less remote. I am not talking about the odd sale of indifferent craft work but about establishing as an institutional side line a service which has genuine social currency. Few people when offered a game of squash, fresh trout for supper or a visit to a mental hospital will choose the latter, so reduce and confuse the choice.

Building needs within hospitals have never allowed courts, sports halls, swimming pools, outdoor pitches or bowling greens to be given any priority, although some do exist. The desirability of patients using facilities outside the hospital has precluded any current expenditure; in any case life-style can rarely compete with life-saving in the allocation of limited resources.

However, children may be better educated about and accepting of psychological disorders if their contact with institutions is made in the context of sharing facilities rather than of providing service. A rising awareness of health and fitness amongst the adult population has created a demand for new sports facilities and the development of leisure centres. Increasing unemployment has created a climate in which money spent on leisure is well justified. Strategies governing public expenditure do not have to divide the healthy from the unhealthy, the barriers that are being slowly broken down might be demolished faster by developing community recreation facilities within the diminishing psychiatric hospitals.

Mobile day centres and support clubs for those with a history of psychiatric disorders recognise the desirability of using unstigmatised facilities, for example church and school halls and a variety of other public buildings. The same wisdom needs to be applied to the 'inward flow' with positive efforts to develop the evening and weekend use of psychiatric units by community groups and organisations. The administrators' cries that any revenue gained would not balance the cost of domestic and security staff should be strongly countered with the argument that social change is a better long-term investment than a piece of sophisticated equipment which will become outdated.

Many institutions have a tradition of producing hand-made items and for including sheltered work within the routine of many patients. Such activities have tended to be cut back as priority has been given to domestic and social rehabilitation and to resettlement. The population remaining within institutions, many of whom are elderly, do not constitute a capable work force — and why should they? Within the community the trend is away from the provision of sheltered or segregated work, even though some long-stay patients who have been resettled may lack a structured routine to their day. The whole question or providing protected, and probably uneconomic, work is fraught with political and ideological arguments. The institution as a 'workhouse' for the destitute is likely to be perceived as a regressive rather than a progressive concept. There is a thin dividing line, which may be viewed differently by therapists, patients, trades unionists and administrators, between providing a service and exploiting those whom you seek to serve. Your opinion must be based on local conditions and the needs of a wide range of people. A sound project is one which provides hospitalised patients with an interesting and stimulating style of life involving contact with people; which provides a supportive and active structure for those rehabilitated patients who are unemployed and at risk of isolation or deterioration; and which engages the general public in an informed and informal contact with psychiatric services.

There is as much need and opportunity for originality and enterprise within the remains of institutions as outside. What is both possible and desirable depends on the needs and tastes of the population and the resources at your disposal. Make a cool appraisal of the entire situation; manufacturing is the option traditionally favoured but it scores low on community involvement. The keeping of livestock also has a tradition but it could well be brought up to date. Free range eggs may have their attractions but the problem experienced by most families is what to do with pet animals when they go away. Short-term admissions for dogs, cats, rabbits or budgerigars, with guaranteed affection and exercise, has much stronger community appeal. To the determined therapist the conversion of the greenery fronting the main entrance to a trout farm has considerable potential. Your own ideas may be less bizarre but it is essential to be positive about institutions in the future, to include them in our overall strategic thinking and to work towards their 'rehabilitation'.

BIBLIOGRAPHY

Bennett D 1978 Community psychiatry. British Journal of Psychiatry 132: 209–220
King's Fund Centre 1984 Seminar report: Health authority joint finance for housing associations.

RECOMMENDED READING

Goldberg D, Huxley P 1980 Mental illness in the community. Tavistock, London

Social Services Committee Enquiry 1984 Community care with special reference to the adult mentally ill and mentally handicapped. British Journal of Occupational Therapy 47(12): 376–377

Walker J K 1986 Out into the community (Casson Memorial Lecture). British Journal of Occupational Therapy 49(5): 144–146

Wing J K, Olsen R 1979 Community care for the mentally disabled. Oxford University Press, Oxford

Wolfensburger W 1972 Principles of normalisation in human services. National Institute on Mental Retardation, Toronto

SOURCES OF INFORMATION

Centre on Environment for the Handicapped
126 Albert Street
London NW1 7NF

Good Practices in Mental Health
380–385 Harrow Road
London W9 2HU

Personal Social Services Research Unit
Cornwallis Building
The University
Canterbury
Kent CT2 7NF

Evaluation of individual
  progress
Evaluation of a method
  of treatment

Principles of simple
  research
The language
The mechanics

12

Evaluation

This book has been written, so far, on the tacit assumption that occupational therapy is a valued and effective service to long-term psychiatric patients. It may be true that the provision of occupational therapy is a manifestation of social compassion, and that it contributes to the self-development and satisfying life-style of disabled people. Such justifications are, however, based on emotion rather than on evidence and may lack power within the systems through which resources are allocated.

The world, as we know it, combines advanced scientific and technical knowledge with developing philosophies of human values and with an economic recession. These three factors co-exist uneasily. Occupational therapy has to justify its practices in terms of quality of life, which is mainly abstract concept, and in terms of efficiency and cost effectiveness, which can be measured.

Occupational therapy is not a commercial enterprise; there is no marketable product. Financial feasibility is based on the savings which can be made through employing our services being greater than the savings which could be made through dispensing with them.

Any profession which bases its practices on tradition rather than on empirical knowledge is particularly vulnerable.

Knowledge and related techniques are continually developing and changing. The 'discrete body of knowledge' which is claimed as central to any practice is made of chewing gum and not of rock. Inadequate theories and ineffective practices have to be identified and discarded at the same rate that new ideas and measures are being developed and tested.

All these concerns contribute to the fact that the evaluation of what has been done is as essential to any practitioner as the assessment of what should be done. Although this responsibility is shared throughout the profession, there are different levels at which investigations can be made. Three levels are described here, although they are not mutually exclusive. These are the evaluation of individual progress, the evaluation of a method of treatment and the principles of simple research.

EVALUATION OF INDIVIDUAL PROGRESS

This is the simplest level of critical investigation but is perhaps the most unreliable. Since one is examining the effects of intervention on one individual there is no control for comparison and a limited opportunity to account for extraneous reasons for improvement or for deterioration. These problems do not outweigh the ethical and practical merits of formalizing, as far as possible, such routine evaluations. Quite simply, if you do not stop and attempt to measure the benefit to the patient of his treatment, that treatment could continue, in an unmodified form, indefinitely.

The key to being able to examine progress lies in the setting of goals at the planning stage. If goals are set which state the criteria for success within a given time, then the moment arrives to decide whether the target has been reached or not. If the goal has been met then this indicates, but does not prove, the effectiveness of treatment. If the goal has not been reached this signals the need to re-examine the methods being used and to adjust the programme, the environment or the style of management accordingly.

A part of evaluation on this level is the acceptance of responsibility for your own knowledge, skills and time. These are resources for which every employed professional is personally accountable. This means having to examine each element of your own performance, identifying strengths and weaknesses and initiating changes towards greater effectiveness. Such changes may include, for example, studying to remedy inadequate knowledge, adjusting routines to make the best use of time, and creating more useful relationships with patients or colleagues. To an extent these responsibilities can be met through the setting of personal goals as described earlier. But it is also essential to appraise with honesty one's own contribution to each activity or relationship.

EVALUATION OF A METHOD OF TREATMENT

To find out whether a method of treatment is effective it needs to be analysed, interpreted and eventually compared with other methods of treatment, or with the absence of treatment. This brings such studies into the realm of comparative research. This section has, however, been included since descriptive, comparative or experimental studies may be the first and most significant venture of students or newly qualified staff who want to improve their own standards of practice.

With a research project the population under study is clearly defined and, if appropriate, a randomly selected representative sample is chosen. Factors which may influence the results, such as age, sex, diagnostic category and duration of treatment are controlling factors. Groups which are being compared within a study are matched as far as possible. The number of groups depends on the complexity of the study, but one group, the control, should always be experiencing no change, or as little change as possible, to their normal routine during the study. The minimum number of groups is, therefore, two — the experimental group consisting of those who are receiving the treatment being evaluated and the control group. If for example, the use of drama is being compared with the use of art then three groups are required.

The next thing to decide is what aspects of the patient's condition or behaviour will be identified, compared at different stages and used as a criterion for success. if factors such as height, weight or intelligence which can be measured are used, this provides quantitative information. It is, however, more likely that qualitative information will be relevant to the occupational therapist. Qualitative information includes features which a number of people may have in common, such as red hair, a place of origin, the ability to dress themselves and their level of social competence. Qualities are often expressed in terms of percentages or ratios within a given group.

A method of identifying quantity or quality is next required. Quantity is usually straightforward since precise tools are available such as tape measures and thermometers. Quality can be uncomplicated to assess, for example counting the number of redheads, or can require more sophisticated methods. Personal independence, span of concentration, dexterity, social competence or self-esteem, for example, all need the development of valid and reliable forms of assessment. It may be necessary to search through existing literature, or to contact others, to find a relevant method which can be used. Otherwise, the means of assessment must be developed and tested before the comparative study can be embarked upon.

Having recorded the existing features or abilities of all members of each group, the active phase can begin. If the effectiveness of treatment is under review, this is likely to be a longitudinal study; that is, one in which the progress of a group is followed through from start to finish.

A cross-sectional study would draw information at one particular time from people who were at different stages, for example investigating the amount of contact with relatives after 1 year, 5 years and 10 years of continuous institutional care respectively.

At predetermined intervals, each group is reassessed. Changes within each group are noted and the degree of changes which has taken place compared between the groups. Minor variations are inevitable and may not mean much; the problem is to decide how great the difference should be before it can be regarded as evidence that the treatment given is responsible for this change. This is where tests of statistical significance become important. A statistician should be able to provide advice about the number of people who should be included in a study and how they should be selected in order to make it valid, and about the tests which can be applied to results in order to give them credibility.

PRINCIPLES OF SIMPLE RESEARCH

The language

The last section included a limited number of examples of the terms used in research. These included control groups, quantitative and qualitative information and longitudinal and cross-sectional studies. The chapter on assessment referred to validity, reliability, different types of variable and statistical significance. It is difficult to introduce the topic of research without becoming involved in the construction of a glossary. However, it is important to be able to read research papers and to use guidelines, written by experienced research workers, for planning your own work. There are, for example, a number of different types of research.

Descriptive research refers to the collection of information about an existing situation and does not involve the researcher in changing or manipulating either events or the environment in any way. Examples could be discovering and recording the percentage of patients who learnt how to dress themselves in hospital and who continue to do so at home, the time spent by basic grade occupational therapists in direct contact with patients, or what the ratio of male to female patients has been in the last year within the domestic training programme.

Comparative research may be based on ideas which arise from noting differences between groups of patients or methods of treatment. The researcher attempts to identify the consequences of these differences. The usual method is to carry out longitudinal or cross-sectional studies. The purpose is to examine existing differences rather than to introduce new methods or to manipulate the environment.

Experimental research is the type of study which involves the direct testing of hypotheses by manipulating the environment or introducing techniques and measuring the results. For example, one could hypothesise that half-day attendance in industrial therapy was as effective, for each patient, as full attendance or that teaching mentally handicapped children to

swim will increase their ability to skip. The experimenter identifies a problem, proposes a hypothesis for its solution and
then manipulates events or the environment to find out
whether he is right or not.

The mechanics

The following processes may be involved at different stages
of carrying out a research project:

Deciding what to investigate

There are so many anomalies and practices that merit investigation that basic ideas should not be a problem. Reading
accounts of other people's research can help to trim ideas
down into specific questions. The most common mistake is
to choose too broad an area of study. For example 'the use
of drama in psychiatry' would be a study almost without
boundaries; 'the value of role-playing exercises to decrease
antisocial behaviour in chronically impaired male patients'
could be a better bet.

Finding out what is already known

Searches within existing literature should at first be broadly
related to the problem and then narrowed down to the
specific investigation you have in mind. There may be several
different theoretical approaches or attitudes applied to the
problem by others. In making use of some and choosing to
reject others it is necessary to give reasons for such decisions.
It may be interesting to repeat a study which has already been
done in order to compare the results.

Designing a hypothesis

This tentative solution should suggest a relationship between
two or more factors, for example between physical exercise
and the degree of confusion experienced by elderly patients
or between attendance at a day centre and readmission to
hospital. If a theoretical frame of reference is being used or
a specific method of treatment, these should be defined. A

piece of descriptive research may not need a hypothesis but may, on completion, suggest relationships which can later be tested.

Designing the study

First decide whether it is descriptive, whether it compares existing systems or whether it carries out experimental tests of new ideas. Whatever the decision it now becomes impossible to put off thinking about variables any longer (see Ch. 7). Note that independent variables may be described in other texts as manipulated variables and that dependent variables also travel under the guise of criterion variables.

Once you have determined the type of study and the variables which are involved then it should be possible to identify what information you require in order to test the hypothesis or to document the existing situation. This information may need to be collected from records, from physiological or psychological testing, from observation or from asking people questions.

Collecting information

Information may be quantitative or qualitative, but in either case it must be reliable. Medical records can be a useful source of quantative information but do not forget that reports of behaviour, and even diagnosis, can be subjective material, particularly when contributed by a large number of people. Interviews may be either structured or less structured in style. A structured interview is one in which the questioner follows a list of questions, each of which has a limited range of responses (like yes/no). This is a bit like acting as a human questionnaire form, with the option of prompting or providing explanations when necessary. A less structured interview allows greater freedom to the respondent to explore the topic. This may be more appropriate if you are collecting information about attitudes or perceptions but provides a greater headache in processing the results.

Observation is useful as long as all the 'observers' are looking for the same thing and applying the same criteria to what they see. A problem can arise if the presence of the observer affects the behaviour of those who are being observed. For this reason observers are often disguised, not necessarily as trees but as participants in other activites or as staff without specific concerns in what is happening.

Questionnaires have to be carefully constructed to avoid ambiguities or irrelevances and should be tested carefully before being given a wide distribution. They may also have a variable, and sometimes disappointing, rate of return. On the other hand they are straightforward to process if properly designed and can give the researcher access to a wider range of people than other methods.

Standardized tests can be used to record physiological states and psychological functions such as attention, memory, orientation and speed of response. Scales for rating person- ality are also available, although these are subject to manip- ulation by the subject.

There are a number of other recognized ways of obtaining information; those mentioned above are examples which may be particularly attractive to occupational therapists. The infor- mation obtained is only valuable if the sample of subjects has been selected correctly. That is, if enough people are involved to make the results valid and if extraneous variables have been eliminated or neutralised.

Organisation of results

Data collected needs to be organised to supply information which can be read by others. Results may be displayed in tables, figures such as bar charts, graphs and other diagrams, or by ranking. Short narrative passages can also clarify information.

At this point, reference books start referring to statistical terms such as means, modes, medians, standard deviations and probabilities. It is true that expert advice is required by most people but some basic appreciation of the language is almost a prerequisite to seeking advice. A mean score is the average; the mode is the score which appears most frequently; the median is the middle point above and below which scores are equally divided. If you imagine a curve of normal distribution for the height of men, these three figures should be easy to calculate. Furthermore this group deviates from the mean both upwards and downwards. Standard deviation is the part of such a curve which includes all those who should be considered as falling within a 'normal' range each way. The range of the first standard deviation includes 68.2% of all individuals, and the range of the second includes 95.4% of the sample.

'Probability' refers to the extent to which differences in results of tests could be due to chance or could be evidence of a causative effect. Several statistical tests, such as the Chi-square and the t-test, can be applied to results to determine their significance. The result of the appropriate statistical tests indicates the level of the probability that the results of the experiment were due to chance. The 99% level of significance is often chosen as the determining level; thus if results achieve this, then there is a less then 1% probability that they were due to chance and are therefore due to some other reason.

Descriptions of how to apply these tests appear in the texts given as recommended reading for this chapter.

This section is not intended to provide all the information required in order to carry out a research project. Its inclusion is intended to show that evaluative studies are within the scope of any occupational therapist.

If we wish to make a positive contribution to the treatment of long term psychiatric patients, or of any other group of disabled people, we have to identify relevant theoretical knowledge, perfect and apply professional skills within treatment and evaluate the results in order to extend the range of available knowledge.

RECOMMENDED READING

Andrews K 1979 Research and the therapist. British Journal of Occupational Therapy 42(2): 44–45

Berry R 1978 How to write a research paper. Pergamon Press, Oxford

Castle W M 1976 Statistics in small doses. Churchill Livingstone, Edinburgh

Hoinville G, Jowell R et al 1977 Survey research and practice. Heinemann, London

Leonard J M 1971 Statistics the arithmetic of decision making. Hodder and Stoughton, London

Notter L E 1979 Essentials of nursing research, 2nd edn. Tavistock, London

Oppenheimer A N 1966 Questionnaire design and attitude measurement. Heinemann, London

Partridge C, Barnitt R 1986 Research guidelines a handbook for therapists. Heinemann, London
Sainsbury P, Kreitman N 1975 Methods of psychiatric research, 2nd edn. Oxford University Press, London
Smith M E 1979 Becoming involved in research. British Journal of Occupational Therapy 42(3): 65–66

Index